Of course, the author welcomes feedback and suggestions for improvement.

Created with love and Affinity Publisher on a Mac.

1st Edition, 2025

Print: Libri Plureos GmbH, Friedensallee 273, 22763 Hamburg

ISBN: 9783692110035

Markus Schall

THE UNCONVENTIONAL HEMORRHOID BOOK

Surviving Hemorrhoid Hell – **and Finding the Way Out**

M. Schall Verlag

https://schall-verlag.de

Table of Contents

PART 1: Invisible but Painful

PART 3: What Might Really Be Behind Hemorrhoids

PART 4: Paths to Relief - What Helps in the Long Run

1 2 3 4 5 6 7 8 9 10 11 12 13 14 15 16 A

Part 1: Invisible but Painful – The Long-Overlooked Common Condition

Chapter 1 – A Hidden Beginning

Hemorrhoids rarely appear overnight. They develop slowly – quietly, inconspicuously, often without pain, sometimes with nothing more than a fleeting moment of irritation that's easy to dismiss. For many, the story begins with a small red spot on the toilet paper. Hardly noticed, hardly ever talked about. And that's exactly what makes them so deceptive: their subtlety is their greatest ally.

It was the same for me. I still remember that first trace of blood – I must have been 15 or 16 years old. At the time, I blamed it on hard stools or a brief irritation. I had no idea that this tiny drop would be the first sign of something that would accompany me for decades. In **Section 1.1**, I talk about exactly that: this first moment – and how I perceived it, or rather, how I ignored it.

Section 1.2 deals with hesitation. Because what I experienced is true for many: the threshold for seeking medical help for discomfort in the anal area is very high. Too high. The reasons vary – from shame to uncertainty to a simple lack of knowledge. In this part, I try to give a voice to this silence and to show why it is so widespread.

Section 1.3 focuses on the quiet progression. I describe how, over the years, I developed a condition that was always "just about bearable" – and how we can get used to symptoms without even realizing it. It's a gradual process in which the unusual eventually becomes the norm. And that is precisely what makes hemorrhoids such a persistent issue.

Finally, in **Section 1.4**, I reflect on why I waited so long to take action – and what I would do differently today. It's not a reproach to my younger self, but an honest look at the patterns many people carry within them: avoidance, endurance, delay. Only in hindsight do these patterns become visible – and offer the chance to learn from them.

So this first chapter is more than just an introduction to the topic. It is a personal reflection. And it is an invitation to every reader to ask themselves: How do I deal with the signals my body sends me – especially the ones no one likes to talk about?

1.1 – Blood in the Stool – My First Encounter with Hemorrhoids

It wasn't a dramatic moment. No emergency, no panic, no pain. Just a little bit of blood. And to be honest, not even for the first time. I was around 15 or 16 years old when I consciously noticed it: a faint red smear on the toilet paper, a single drop in the water – nothing more. Nothing to worry about, I thought at the time.

Like many others at that age, I dismissed it right away. Blood? Oh well. Maybe a small scratch. Maybe from straining. Or a hard bowel movement. Surely there was some harmless explanation. What it definitely couldn't be – I was convinced – was something that needed to be discussed. Least of all with a doctor.

Back then, anything related to the bowels was, for me – and probably for many other teenagers – a private realm. Not just physically, but emotionally too. Nothing that happened "down there" felt like something to share. It was a personal matter. And as long as life carried on and there was no real pain, there was no reason to question anything.

A Subtle, Lingering Problem Over the Years

In the years that followed, the issue became an occasional recurrence. Not constant, but not a one-off either. It felt as though my body was gently trying to tell me, "Something's not right." And I? I simply didn't listen. In hindsight, that's probably one of the most common mistakes in dealing with hemorrhoids – not the symptoms themselves, but the months or even years of ignoring them.

For me, it was a gradual process: the occasional bleeding slowly became more frequent. In my twenties, it became increasingly common to see traces of blood after a bowel movement. At first, I told myself: Maybe you sat too long. Maybe you didn't drink enough water. Maybe you haven't been eating enough vegetables. But even small lifestyle changes didn't lead to real improvement.

The bleeding was never heavy – but it was persistent. And most of all: It was disturbingly consistent. Today, when I talk to others, I realize how many men have had similar experiences – but almost no one talks about them. For many, blood in the stool feels like a sign of weakness, a kind of stigma one carries in silence. Yet this is exactly where openness would help most.

Better Late Than Never – Taking Responsibility

Still, nearly fifteen years passed before I saw a specialist for the first time. I was in my early thirties by then. The bleeding was no longer just "occasional" – it had become an almost daily companion. Sometimes just a trace, sometimes clearly visible. And yet it took until I reached a point where I could no longer ignore it – and no longer wanted to.

What finally prompted me was my father. He brought up the topic – calmly, without pressure. I believe he had had similar experiences himself and wanted to help me before things got worse. I remember how I resisted inside – not out of defiance, but because I was ashamed. I was young, healthy, had no chronic conditions. And now I was supposed to get help "down there"? It felt like admitting to something I couldn't even name.

Today, I see it very differently. It wasn't an admission of weakness – it was the first step toward taking responsibility. But that step came late – and the path leading up to it was marked by ignorance, uncertainty, and the instinctive urge to suppress rather than understand.

If I could offer one piece of advice today – to young people, or older ones alike – it would be this: Take your body seriously when it sends you signals. And above all: Talk about it.

What seems like a small issue can grow over the years – not just physically, but emotionally too. And there are ways to address it early. But they always begin with the courage to take a closer look.

1.2 – Why So Many People Wait Too Long

Hemorrhoids are a widespread condition – yet a very quiet one. According to estimates, between 50 and 70 percent of all adults experience enlarged hemorrhoids or related rectal issues at some point in their lives. And yet the topic remains largely invisible in everyday life. It is not discussed, not shared, not questioned. Instead, a collective silence prevails – a silence that harms many because it leads them to act too late, or not at all.

The reasons for this are complex. Some are cultural, others psychological. And of course, personal experiences and fears also play a role.

1. The Barrier of Shame Is Deep

There are few parts of the body that people are less willing to talk about than the anus. While back pain, stomach issues, or even incontinence are now discussed more openly, hemorrhoids remain a taboo topic – even in the 21st century. For many, the idea of telling someone about itching, bleeding, or a noticeable bulge around the anus is deeply embarrassing – even when speaking to a doctor.

This is especially true for men. The societal pressure to "function" without showing any weakness often extends into the most private areas. The fear of undressing for a proctological exam – of being literally and figuratively "exposed" – is not to be underestimated.

2. The Symptoms Are Gradual – and Easy to Ignore

Hemorrhoids typically develop slowly. In the early stages, the symptoms are usually mild: an occasional burning, itching, or light traces of blood on the toilet paper. Nothing that really hurts. And above all: nothing that seems immediately limiting. That's what makes the problem so tricky.

Because the discomfort doesn't seem urgent, it's easy to push the issue aside. Many think, "It'll go away on its own," or, "It's probably just from straining." This mindset is human – but dangerous. Left untreated, hemorrhoids can grow, become inflamed, or turn chronic. What starts as a minor irritation can become a major issue.

I experienced this gradual progression over many years. There was no sudden deterioration – just a slow shift from "barely noticeable" to "constantly present." And because it happened so gradually, I barely noticed the change – until I realized I had already accepted the condition as "normal."

3. Lack of Knowledge and Downplaying the Problem

Another reason many people hesitate is simply: lack of knowledge. We learn little to nothing about the topic in school. It's rarely discussed among friends. Many people don't even know what hemorrhoids really are – let alone when to take action.

To make matters worse, many general practitioners react cautiously or don't take symptoms like itching or bleeding seriously enough. Proper information and education are often lacking. This reinforces the feeling that it's not worth doing anything – at least not yet.

4. Fear of the Examination

The fear of being examined is also a major factor – especially when it comes to a proctological evaluation. For many, the idea of undergoing such an exam feels like a loss of control. The position on the exam chair is unfamiliar, intimate, and possibly uncomfortable.

On top of that, there are many myths about how painful or humiliating such procedures supposedly are. In reality, most proctologists today are experienced, kind, and professional. But this knowledge often comes only after someone has finally worked up the courage to go.

Conclusion: Silence Prolongs Suffering

There are many reasons why people wait too long when dealing with hemorrhoids. Shame, insecurity, lack of information, and fear blend into a deep inner resistance that's hard to overcome. That's why it's so important to talk about this topic – calmly, respectfully, without mockery or exaggeration. The earlier you act, the greater the chance that a simple change in daily habits – such as diet, exercise, or using a cream – will be enough. And the longer you wait, the more likely it becomes that surgery will be necessary.

Looking back, I wish I had taken action sooner. Not because it would have been easier – but because it was unnecessary to suffer in silence for so many years. But like with so many others, the pressure to act only grew once the symptoms could no longer be ignored.

The path to improvement almost always begins with a simple sentence:

"I think something's not quite right – I'm going to take a look."

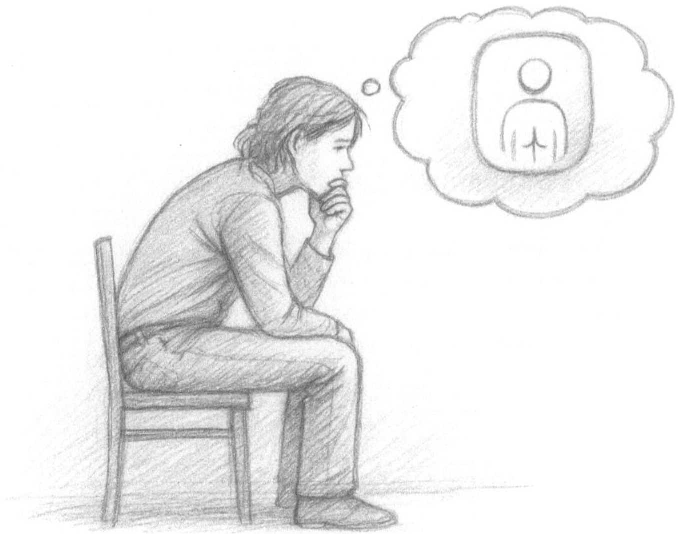

1.3 – The Silent Progression Over Many Years

Hemorrhoids are rarely a sudden catastrophe. They don't begin with a sharp pain that startles you or with a dramatic symptom that forces immediate action. Instead, their course is often so gradual that they aren't even recognized as a condition for many years – just an occasional nuisance, somehow normal, a background noise of everyday life. That's what makes them so insidious.

It was the same for me.

After noticing the first traces of blood around the age of 15 or 16, it remained an occasional episode for a long time. Nothing that disrupted my day. No pain, no itching, no sensation of something being "off" – just a bit of blood on the toilet paper now and then. Sometimes nothing for weeks, then a few days where it was more noticeable. I got used to it, even if unintentionally.

What I didn't know at the time: even this early stage could have been classified as grade 1 hemorrhoids – a phase in which tissue in the anal area is already changing, but hasn't yet become enlarged or prolapsed. At this stage, hemorrhoids are generally easy to treat and, in some cases, can even regress through simple lifestyle adjustments. But that requires recognition – and acceptance.

I did neither.

Normalization as a Coping Strategy

Instead, what once seemed unusual gradually became "normal." A little blood? Just part of the routine. Maybe something spicy I ate. Maybe I didn't drink enough water. Maybe just a hard stool. There was always a harmless explanation – sometimes sincerely believed, sometimes just an excuse to avoid thinking about it any further.

This kind of normalization is common with many chronic issues – not just hemorrhoids. People have an amazing ability to adapt as long as something doesn't feel acutely threatening. The pain doesn't have to disappear – it just needs to be predictable. And if symptoms remain small enough not to disrupt daily life, they eventually fade into the background.

And so the years passed.

Slow but Steady

In my twenties, the episodes became more frequent. What had been occasional bleeding turned into a regular occurrence. It no longer happened every few weeks – sometimes several times a week, later almost daily. Other symptoms began to appear slowly: a slight pressure when sitting, a vague itching, especially in the evenings, sometimes a sense of tightness – not painful, but noticeable. None of it was dramatic or clearly defined – but taken together, it began to erode my quality of life.

I could still exercise. I sat at a desk for hours each day. I drove, went to the movies, lived a completely normal life. But in the background, something was always there. A quiet irritation. A sense that something wasn't quite right. And again: I didn't talk to anyone about it.

The Fine Line Between Everyday Life and a Real Problem

It wasn't until my early thirties – about 15 years after the first signs – that I reached a point where I could no longer ignore it. The daily bleeding had become a burden. The symptoms were clearer, the uncertainty greater. Most of all, there was a growing inner alarm. A quiet but persistent discomfort that said: "This isn't normal anymore."

What I didn't know back then – but understand much better now – is that advanced hemorrhoids aren't just a physical issue; they affect your mental well-being too. Living with an "invisible" condition that you can't really explain and that no one else sees can change how you view yourself. You begin to lose some trust in your body – and sometimes in yourself.

Why the Progression Often Goes Unnoticed – or Gets Ignored

Many people experience a very similar course. And almost everyone I've spoken to about it later said the same thing at some point: "It kind of crept up on me." That's the key. The progression is too slow to trigger alarm – but too consistent to be harmless.

And let's be honest: most of us would rather not look too closely. Focusing on your anal health forces you to deal with topics that lie far outside the comfort zone. Hygiene, control, intimacy, shame – it all plays a role. So we prefer to suppress the issue instead of confronting the possible causes or seeking a clear diagnosis. At least for as long as we still can.

Conclusion: If You Don't Look, You May Look Too Late

The progression of hemorrhoids is, in many cases, not a medical drama but a psychological pattern. It starts out harmless, continues quietly, gets ignored – and slowly but steadily develops further. Only when the suffering becomes too much do we begin to seek help.

Looking back, I would say this: My body gave me very clear signals early on. I just didn't take them seriously. Not out of recklessness or pride – but out of a mix of uncertainty, lack of knowledge, and the wish not to deal with this part of my body at all.

But eventually, the body forces you to confront it. And in retrospect, I'm grateful that this process didn't happen suddenly, but – in the truest sense – step by step. Because it helped me understand later just how multi-layered this development was – and how important it is to start paying attention early on.

1.4 – A Personal Reflection: How I Reacted Too Late

There are things in life you only truly see in hindsight – with a clarity you wish you'd had back then. Hemorrhoids, for me, definitely fall into that category. It's not that I didn't notice something was wrong. On the contrary – my body gave me clear signals over many years. But I didn't take them seriously. Or, to be more precise: I didn't want to take them seriously.

Looking back now, my response to the first symptoms – the blood in the stool, the slight itching, the growing sensation of pressure – was one big internal shrug. Somewhere deep down, I knew it wasn't ideal. But I wasn't in pain, I could work, sleep, travel, live. And as long as the discomfort wasn't severe, it didn't feel like a "real" problem. I simply adjusted to it – without ever really deciding to.

Maybe that's exactly what so many people in similar situations do: a quiet inner agreement with a condition that really should be treated. Not out of laziness. Not out of ignorance. But simply because the body still "works." Because there's no external pressure to act. Because the topic is embarrassing. And because we'd rather go to the doctor for anything else – just not this.

A Topic You Don't Want to Open

I've never been someone easily alarmed by doctors or diagnoses. I've always observed things closely and questioned a lot on my own. But in this case, that very tendency led me to rationalize everything. If there was blood in the stool, it was just from a hard bowel movement. If there was itching, it was just irritated tissue. There was always some explanation that made it easier to postpone the issue until tomorrow. And then until the day after. And at some point, you simply get used to it.

Add to that the usual mix of shame, uncertainty, and resistance: who wants to see a proctologist? It's not like going to the dentist or orthopedist. This is about a part of your body you hardly ever see yourself – and that you're even less willing to show someone else.

It feels vulnerable, almost humiliating. Especially as a man, especially when you're otherwise healthy, active, in the middle of life. A "rectal problem" just doesn't fit into that self-image.

So I waited. And kept on waiting.

The Moment I Couldn't Look Away Any Longer

Only when the symptoms became a daily companion – the bleeding, the tightness, the constant feeling that something "down there" wasn't right – did the realization slowly begin to form: This can't go on.

But even then, it wasn't my own motivation that pushed me to act.

It was my father who finally brought it up – gently, without pressure, but with a clear message: "You should have that checked out." I don't think he meant it only medically, but also for the sake of my inner balance. He had probably seen how much the issue was affecting me emotionally – even though I had never spoken openly about it.

At first, I was almost offended. Not because he was wrong – but because I felt caught. It was as if someone had opened the door to a room I'd kept closed for years. And for that very reason, it was the right moment.

I did go to the doctor – much later than I should have. And yes, the diagnosis confirmed that I could have received help years earlier. But I don't regret the path I took. Because it showed me just how many layers are involved in a process like this – not just physical ones, but emotional ones too. Not just symptoms, but also the images we carry of ourselves – of weakness, illness, control.

Today I Know: "Too Late" Is Still Not "Too Late"

I hesitated for a long time. I reacted too late. But I did react. And that counts.

What I wish – for my younger self and for others today – is not a perfect way of dealing with symptoms, but a culture in which people take themselves seriously sooner. A culture in which it's normal to talk to a doctor about blood in the stool. One where people don't wait years until their quality of life noticeably declines. And where even men can openly say:

"I've got a problem – and I want to understand it."

Because in the end, that's where every solution begins.

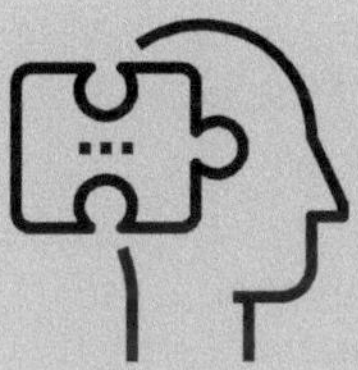

Did You Know…?

Everyone has hemorrhoids – they are a natural cushion of blood vessels located in the lower rectum. Problems only arise when these cushions become enlarged or inflamed. Many people live for years without noticing their enlarged hemorrhoids.

Chapter 2 – Understanding the Body: A Foundation for Clarity

Before diving into causes, treatment options, and personal experiences related to hemorrhoids, it's worth starting with the basics: the human body itself. Many misunderstandings, fears, or unnecessary worries arise simply from a lack of knowledge about what's happening in the rectal area. And that's not meant as a criticism – this part of the body is rarely discussed in school, daily life, or even in medical contexts beyond the surface level.

Yet especially in such a sensitive area, it is incredibly helpful to understand – calmly and factually – what's actually going on when hemorrhoids become noticeable, and how to recognize them in the first place.

In **Section 2.1**, we explore the anatomy of the rectum – in other words: what exactly is going on down there. We'll take a look at how the body controls the closing of the anus, the role hemorrhoidal cushions play in that process, and why this vascular tissue actually serves an important function. Once you understand that hemorrhoids are not initially a disease but a natural part of the body, it becomes much easier to approach the topic with calm and clarity.

Section 2.2 focuses on the distinction between internal and external hemorrhoids. Many people confuse these terms or mix them up with entirely different conditions. Here we explain where the boundary lies, what typical symptoms look like, and how treatment approaches differ depending on the type.

Section 2.3 is devoted to the so-called severity levels. Medicine divides hemorrhoidal disease into four stages – from barely noticeable early signs to a permanent prolapse that may require surgical intervention. This classification helps not only doctors but also patients to better understand their own situation – and to develop realistic expectations for treatment.

The final section of this **chapter, 2.4**, covers other rectal conditions that are often mistaken for hemorrhoids. These include anal vein thrombosis, anal fissures, or harmless skin tags known as marisques – but also more serious diagnoses such as fistulas or tumors. This overview is meant to help readers better understand common symptoms and recognize when a medical evaluation is especially important.

2.1 – Anatomy: What's Going On Down There

Anyone dealing with hemorrhoids – whether personally affected or simply curious – can't avoid a brief anatomical overview. Only by understanding how the body functions in this area can we grasp why symptoms occur – and how to manage them effectively. The good news: it's not rocket science. The anatomy of the rectum is complex, but logically organized. And above all, it serves one key purpose: control.

The Rectum – More Than Just the "Last Section"

The rectum (medically: rectum) is the final part of the human digestive tract. It measures about 12 to 15 centimeters in length and begins where the large intestine ends. Its main function is to store stool – the already dehydrated, "finished" waste material – until the next bowel movement.

What makes the rectum special is its ability to finely regulate this process. While the rest of the intestine is primarily concerned with transport and nutrient absorption, the rectum is all about precision and timing. Together with the brain, it decides when it's the right time to let go. And in this decision, one particular structure plays a crucial role: the hemorrhoidal tissue.

The Hemorrhoidal Cushion – An Important Sealing System

What people commonly refer to as "hemorrhoids" is not necessarily something pathological – at least not in the beginning. Every human being has hemorrhoidal cushions: well-supplied, sponge-like vascular pads located around the anal canal. They sit above the sphincter muscle, are soft and elastic, and – together with the surrounding muscles – form a finely tuned closure mechanism.

You can think of this tissue as a natural seal – somewhat like a rubber gasket in a valve. At rest, the cushion ensures that the rectum is sealed airtight and watertight. During a bowel movement, the cushion compresses and partially empties, temporarily suspending its function – only to refill and reseal afterward.

This function is crucial for fine continence – the ability to consciously retain or release gas, liquid, and solid stool. Without the hemorrhoidal cushions, the sphincter muscle alone would not be able to maintain this level of control.

Double Protection: The Sphincter Muscles

This sealing system is supported by two layers of muscle:

The internal sphincter (musculus sphincter ani internus):

This muscle works involuntarily, without conscious control. It ensures the anus remains closed under normal conditions.

The external sphincter (musculus sphincter ani externus):

This muscle can be consciously contracted – for example, when you want to delay a bowel movement. It can be trained and is often targeted in pelvic floor or postnatal exercises.

Together with the hemorrhoidal cushions, these muscles form a delicate system of reflexes, pressure control, and fine coordination.

When Balance Turns Into a Problem

Hemorrhoids only become a problem when this natural balance is disrupted – for example, by:

- Excessive straining during bowel movements
- Constant pressure in the pelvic area (due to poor posture, pregnancy, or being overweight)
- Weak connective tissue
- Chronic constipation or diarrhea
- Poor diet or dehydration

In such cases, the hemorrhoidal tissue can swell, shift downward, and become permanently enlarged. That's when medicine refers to it as hemorrhoidal disease. The once-healthy cushion has now become a clinical problem.

Location Matters: Internal vs. External Hemorrhoids

"Classic" hemorrhoids are located above the so-called dentate line – a fine boundary inside the anal canal that separates the sensitive outer skin from the less sensitive inner mucosa.

Internal hemorrhoids:

These arise above the dentate line and are often painless because this area contains very few pain receptors. They tend to bleed but rarely cause pain in early stages.

External hemorrhoids:

These develop below the dentate line and are covered by sensitive skin – which is why they can be painful, swollen, itchy, or tender to the touch. What many feel as a "lump near the anus" is often such an external hemorrhoid – or in some cases, an anal vein thrombosis.

An Interplay – Not Just a Single Part

The anatomy around the anus is a finely tuned interaction of muscles, nerves, blood vessels, skin, and mucosa. That's why even small changes – mechanical, inflammatory, or muscular – can throw the system off balance.

Hemorrhoids are not some "quirk of nature" – they are a necessary part of our anatomy. They only become a problem when they enlarge, shift, or become inflamed.

Once you understand that, it becomes easier to face the issue with calm – and with a willingness to address the causes, not just the symptoms.

2.2 – The Difference Between Internal and External Hemorrhoids

When people hear the word "hemorrhoids," they often immediately think of lumps, itching, pain – and something that's felt "on the outside" of the anus. But this picture is often imprecise or even misleading. In medical terms, there is a clear distinction between internal and external hemorrhoids – and these two types differ significantly in origin, location, symptoms, and treatment.

The Anatomical Boundary: The Dentate Line

The most important distinction runs along a line inside the anal canal called the dentate line. It sits about 2 to 3 centimeters inside the anus and marks the boundary between two different types of tissue:

Above the dentate line is mucous membrane tissue (similar to that in the mouth or intestine), which has very few pain receptors.

Below it lies normal, sensitive skin with many nerve endings.

This line determines whether something is painful or not – and whether the condition is classified as internal or external hemorrhoids.

Internal Hemorrhoids – The "Classic" Vascular Cushions

Location and Origin:

Internal hemorrhoids develop above the dentate line. They are part of the natural hemorrhoidal cushion present in every person. In hemorrhoidal disease, these vascular structures become abnormally enlarged, lose elasticity, and gradually begin to prolapse downward.

Typical Symptoms:

- Bright red blood on the stool or toilet paper
- Moist sensation around the anus
- Feeling of incomplete bowel evacuation
- In later stages: bulging tissue felt during straining
- Usually no pain – especially in early stages

Progression by Severity:

Internal hemorrhoids are medically classified into four grades:

- **Grade I**: Enlarged tissue, not visible or palpable
- **Grade II**: Prolapse during straining, retracts on its own
- **Grade III**: Must be manually pushed back in
- **Grade IV**: Permanently prolapsed, cannot be retracted

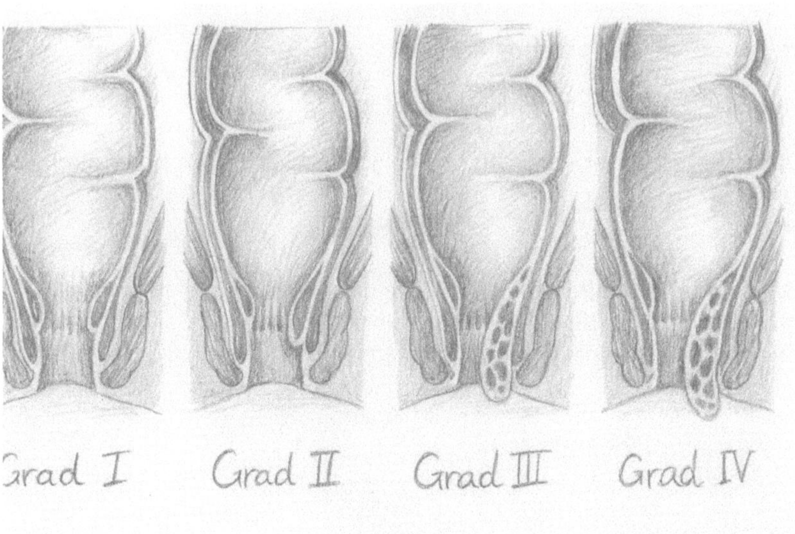

Treatment:

In early stages, conservative treatments are common (ointments, dietary changes, sitz baths). In more advanced cases, procedures like rubber band ligation, infrared coagulation, or surgery may be recommended.

External Hemorrhoids – Often Mistaken for Other Conditions

Location and Origin:

What many people call "external hemorrhoids" are actually changes below the dentate line. Medically speaking, these are not enlarged hemorrhoidal cushions, but rather venous issues or skin changes, such as:

- **Anal vein thromboses** (sudden, very painful lumps)
- **Perianal skin tags** (loose skin flaps after inflammation)
- **Inflamed glands** or small abscesses

Typical Symptoms:

- Sharp, stabbing pain
- Pressure or tension around the anus
- Visible and palpable lumps at the anal margin
- Often sudden onset – e.g., after straining, heavy lifting, or prolonged sitting

Important:

External hemorrhoids almost always cause pain because they occur in a highly sensitive area. Many patients who complain of "hemorrhoids" are actually referring to these external findings – and are surprised when the diagnosis is different.

Treatment:

Common measures include cooling ointments, pain relief, sitz baths, and – in the case of thromboses – minor surgical removal if needed. Proper posture and rest are also important. Surgery is usually only required for recurring or severe cases.

Two Types – Two Approaches

Whether internal or external, both types can cause discomfort – but they differ clearly in appearance, sensation, and treatment strategy.

Internal hemorrhoids tend to be chronic, subtle, and painless – often going unnoticed for a long time.

External changes are usually acute, visible, and painful – often leading people to seek medical help right away.

And What If It's Both?

In practice, many patients have mixed forms. Especially in advanced stages, enlarged internal hemorrhoids can occur alongside irritation or changes in the external area. That's why it's so important to have symptoms professionally examined – even if it feels uncomfortable. Only then can the correct condition be identified and properly treated.

Conclusion: Looking Closely Pays Off

The distinction between internal and external hemorrhoids is more than just academic. It influences treatment options, prognosis – and your personal understanding of your body. Knowing the source of your symptoms helps you respond more effectively and take the right steps.

You don't have to be a medical expert to grasp this. But you should be willing to look at it honestly – especially when it's uncomfortable.

Because good decisions begin with good information.

2.3 – Severity Levels: From Mild Finding to Surgical Indication

Not all hemorrhoids are the same. And not every change is automatically a medical condition. What really matters is how much the natural hemorrhoidal cushions have enlarged, how far they have prolapsed – and whether they return to their original position.

Based on these criteria, hemorrhoidal disease is medically divided into four severity levels. This classification helps not only with diagnosis but also in selecting the right treatment.

Grade I – The Silent Change

The hemorrhoids are slightly enlarged but remain entirely inside the anal canal. They are not visible from the outside and cannot be felt, even during straining. The mucosa covering the tissue is usually intact, though minor bleeding may occur.

Symptoms:

- Bright red blood on toilet paper or in the toilet bowl
- Occasional burning or mild itching
- No sensation of pressure or a foreign body

Treatment:

- No surgery required
- Conservative measures such as a high-fiber diet, adequate hydration, avoiding straining, and over-the-counter creams or suppositories
- In many cases, reversible

Personal Note:

Many people live with grade I hemorrhoids for years – often without even knowing it. My own early signs began during this stage, long before I ever received a diagnosis.

Grade II – The Beginning of Prolapse

The hemorrhoids temporarily protrude from the anal canal during bowel movements but retract on their own afterward. The tissue is clearly enlarged, and elasticity begins to decline.

Symptoms:

- Bleeding during or after bowel movements
- Moist or damp sensation around the anus
- Mild pressure, occasional itching
- First signs of irritation when sitting

Treatment:

Combination of conservative care and minor procedures (e.g., rubber band ligation, infrared coagulation)

Important: initiate lifestyle changes to prevent progression

Note:

At this stage, effective treatment is still relatively straightforward – if addressed early.

Grade III – Manual Repositioning Required

The hemorrhoids prolapse during straining and do not retract on their own. They must be manually pushed back in, which can be uncomfortable or effortful.

Symptoms:

- Heavier bleeding
- Noticeable prolapse during bowel movements
- Frequent pressure or the feeling that "something is in the way"
- Itching, discharge, and in some cases, mild pain

Treatment:

- Conservative methods are often no longer sufficient
- Rubber band ligation, often in multiple sessions, is commonly recommended
- In some cases, surgical procedures (e.g., THD, laser) may be necessary

Personal Experience:

When I finally saw a doctor in 2014, I was diagnosed with a grade III–IV condition. The symptoms had already become chronic. In hindsight, this was the point where more decisive treatment was needed.

Grade IV – Permanent Prolapse

The hemorrhoidal tissue is permanently prolapsed outside the anus and cannot be pushed back in. The tissue is usually visibly altered, often irritated or inflamed, and symptoms are significant.

Symptoms:

- Constant moisture or discharge
- Pain when sitting or walking
- Inflammation and secretion
- Social limitations and ongoing discomfort

Treatment:

- Surgical intervention is usually necessary
- Modern methods aim for tissue-sparing techniques (e.g., laser, THD, stapled hemorrhoidopexy)
- Recovery may take several weeks

Comment:

A grade IV diagnosis doesn't mean "there's nothing that can be done" – but it does require clear and committed action. Even then, it's worth taking a holistic look at posture, diet, and lifestyle.

Transitions and Mixed Forms

The four severity levels provide a helpful framework – but they're not a rigid system. In real life, many patients fall between stages or have combined symptoms, including external findings like anal vein thrombosis or skin tags (marisques) that intensify the discomfort.

A thorough medical examination is therefore essential – not only to determine the exact stage but also to choose the most appropriate treatment.

Early Assessment Makes a Difference

Knowing what stage your condition is in helps you take targeted action – and often achieve significant relief with far less effort.

The most important takeaway: The earlier you act, the better your chances for gentle, non-invasive treatment.

Hemorrhoids are not a life sentence – but they do require attention. And when you understand the different stages, you'll also see:

There are many ways to find relief – if you start early.

2.4 – Other Conditions in the Anal and Rectal Area

When people experience discomfort around the anus or during bowel movements, they often assume it must be hemorrhoids. And indeed, hemorrhoids are the most common cause of symptoms like itching, burning, moisture, or blood on the toilet paper. But they are not the only cause. There are several other conditions in the anal and rectal area that present with similar symptoms – but differ greatly in cause, course, and treatment.

That's why it's worth taking a closer look before self-diagnosing with "hemorrhoids." Not everything that causes symptoms "down there" is actually related to enlarged hemorrhoidal tissue.

Anal Vein Thrombosis – A Sudden, Painful Lump

Anal vein thrombosis is one of the most common "false friends" of hemorrhoids. It's a blood clot in an external vein, just beneath the skin at the edge of the anus. It is often triggered by intense straining, heavy lifting, prolonged sitting, or other mechanical stress.

Typical features:

- Sudden onset of a hard, bluish-colored lump
- Sharp, stabbing pain when sitting, moving, or during bowel movements
- Little to no itching
- No discharge or moisture

Did You Know…?

Many people with hemorrhoids also have an undiagnosed CMD (craniomandibular dysfunction).

Postural imbalances in the jaw and neck area can affect the pelvis through the fascia system.

Treatment:

- Usually harmless but uncomfortable
- Local ointments (e.g. with heparin), cold compresses, rest
- In more severe cases: minor surgical drainage

Difference from hemorrhoids:

Hemorrhoids tend to have a chronic course, while an anal thrombosis appears suddenly and acutely. Patients are often alarmed by the rapid formation of the lump – but it usually heals completely within a few days to weeks.

Anal Fissure – A Small Tear That Hurts a Lot

An anal fissure is a small tear in the sensitive skin lining the anal canal, typically located at the front or back midline. It's often caused by hard stool, excessive straining, or sudden overstretching.

Typical features:

- Intense pain during or just after bowel movements (often sharp or burning)
- Spasms of the sphincter muscle
- Minor bleeding (usually on the toilet paper only)
- May become chronic, with scar tissue formation

Treatment:

- Gentle care, soft stool, anti-inflammatory ointments
- Muscle-relaxing creams (e.g. with diltiazem or nifedipine)
- In chronic cases: surgical removal or minimally invasive procedures

Difference from hemorrhoids:

Fissures cause sharp, well-localized pain, while hemorrhoids tend to cause pressure, itching, or moisture – often without significant pain.

Perianal Skin Tags – Harmless but Sometimes Annoying

Skin tags (also called marisques) are soft folds of skin at the anal margin, often left behind after inflammation, thrombosis, or chronic friction. They are not dangerous but can be cosmetically or hygienically bothersome.

Typical features:

- Soft, often asymmetrical skin protrusions
- No pain or itching – unless inflamed
- Often perceived as a "bothersome flap of skin"
- Rarely associated with embarrassment

Treatment:

- Usually not necessary
- Removal only in case of recurring inflammation or for cosmetic reasons

Difference from hemorrhoids:

Skin tags are skin changes, not vascular issues. They don't bleed, don't cause internal symptoms, and are not considered medically significant.

Perianal Abscesses and Fistulas – Hidden Infections

A perianal abscess is a collection of pus in the tissue around the anus. It usually forms from inflamed glands but can also result from small injuries or infections. Fistulas are chronic tunnels that may develop between the inner rectum and the skin surface – often following an abscess.

Typical features:

- Painful swelling, redness, and tenderness near the anus
- General feeling of illness, possibly mild fever
- Pus discharge or moist, weeping areas
- Recurring inflammation in the case of fistulas

Treatment:

- Usually surgical (incision of the abscess, fistula surgery)
- Antibiotics as a supplement only
- Important: Early diagnosis prevents spread

Difference from hemorrhoids:

Abscesses and fistulas are serious infections, while hemorrhoids are vascular conditions. The symptoms are typically more severe, with stronger pain and general illness signs.

Rectal Tumors and Polyps – Rare, but Important to Know

In rare cases, benign polyps or malignant tumors in the rectum can cause symptoms that resemble hemorrhoids – such as bleeding or pressure.

Warning signs:

- Persistent, often darker bleeding
- Unexplained weight loss
- Alternating diarrhea and constipation
- Unusually frequent urge to defecate

Important:

A thorough examination with endoscopy (e.g. proctoscopy or colonoscopy) is essential. Especially after age 50, unclear symptoms should not automatically be attributed to hemorrhoids.

Conclusion: Not Everything Is What It Seems

Discomfort in the anal area often presents similarly – but the underlying causes can be very different. That's why it's important not to jump to conclusions or treat symptoms with an over-the-counter "hemorrhoid cream" without proper clarification. Knowing the exact cause allows for more targeted – and more effective – treatment.

And even though a visit to the proctologist may feel intimidating, it can save you from unnecessary suffering – especially if the issue isn't hemorrhoids at all, but something else entirely.

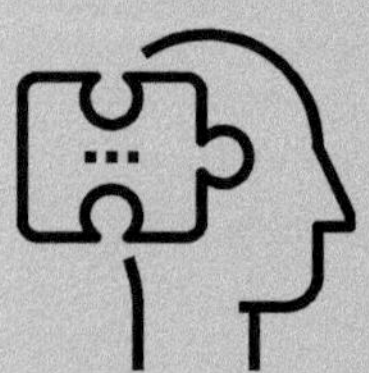

Did You Know…?

Even in hemorrhoid surgery, gentler techniques such as the THD method or laser procedures are increasingly used today – but proper aftercare remains crucial to the success of the treatment.

Chapter 3 – When Discomfort Becomes Everyday Life: Taking Symptoms Seriously Before They Escalate

Many people associate hemorrhoids primarily with a noticeable lump or bleeding during bowel movements. But in reality, the condition often begins much earlier – and in more subtle ways. It starts with small irritations that gradually creep into daily life: a slight itch, a burning sensation that won't go away, a damp feeling that feels out of place, or a vague sense that "something isn't quite right."

It is precisely in these early stages that there is a real chance to stop or ease the progression. But that requires awareness – and the knowledge of which symptoms deserve attention.

This chapter is dedicated to exactly those signs and their typical patterns. It's an invitation to listen more closely – not out of fear, but out of respect for your own body.

In the first **section, 3.1**, we focus on the quiet symptoms: itching, burning, and moisture. These may seem harmless at first glance, but they are often early signs of an imbalance in the anal area – usually caused by irritated hemorrhoidal tissue that can no longer perform its function properly. This initial stage is often overlooked or mistaken for a skin issue. Yet simple measures at this point can already make a big difference.

Section 3.2 addresses the topic of pain during bowel movements or while sitting. Pain is always a warning sign – and especially unpleasant in this area. This section explains how the pain arises, what to watch for, and why it's important not to ignore it or simply cover it up with painkillers.

In **section 3.3**, we focus on a central issue: bleeding. For many, it's the first real cause for concern – and often the moment when they begin to take hemorrhoids seriously. We'll look at when bleeding can be considered harmless, when it should be evaluated, and what it reveals about the condition of the tissue.

Finally, **section 3.4** explores the slow progression: how minor symptoms can turn into a chronic condition over the years, subtly impacting daily life without being fully noticed. This part highlights how many people unknowingly adjust to restrictions – and why it's still worth tuning in to your body, even after a long time.

3.1 – Itching, Burning, and Moisture – An Underestimated Burden

When people think of hemorrhoids, they often picture bleeding or a noticeable lump. What's frequently overlooked, however, are the symptoms that tend to appear first – and that silently but persistently affect daily life: itching, burning, and unpleasant moisture in the anal area. These are symptoms people rarely talk about, partly because they're hard to describe – which makes it all the more important to take a closer look.

When the Anus Itches – More Than Just Skin Irritation

Anal itching is a common symptom. Many experience it as a tingling, pulling, or tickling sensation that comes and goes – and sometimes becomes a constant companion. It's particularly bothersome at night, while resting, or after a bowel movement. The itch can feel so deep that it's hard to localize. And it's often accompanied by shame: scratching your bottom – even internally – just feels "unclean."

But itching is usually not a sign of poor hygiene, but rather an indication of irritated skin or mucosa. In the case of hemorrhoids, it's often caused by enlarged hemorrhoidal tissue that protrudes slightly, secretes mucus, and irritates the delicate skin around the anus. The thin skin at the border between the inner mucosa and the outer environment is especially sensitive.

What follows is a vicious cycle: the itching leads to unconscious scratching or rubbing – during washing, wiping, or even while sleeping. This can cause small injuries, which may become inflamed. The longer it continues, the more the skin changes: it becomes more sensitive, dry, and fragile. The itching persists.

Burning – The Quiet Echo of Irritation

Compared to itching, burning is often less noticeable at first, but more persistent. It typically occurs after a bowel movement or while sitting – especially on hard surfaces or for prolonged periods. Many describe it as a hot, raw, or chafed sensation. Again, the cause is often the slightly prolapsed hemorrhoidal tissue, which leads to subtle changes in the mucosa and makes the area more sensitive.

In addition, continuous moisture can create an anal-eczematous environment: the skin becomes damp, softened, and sore. Similar to diaper rash, inflammation can occur when the skin is constantly irritated and moist. Burning is the body's clearest message that something is out of balance.

Moisture – The Symptom No One Talks About

Moisture is one of the most unpleasant – and most commonly suppressed – symptoms. Many people find it deeply embarrassing, as it is associated with wetness, odor, and a sense of losing control. What often happens is that enlarged hemorrhoids cause small amounts of mucus or moisture to leak from the anal canal – sometimes unnoticed, sometimes experienced as a constant feeling of "being wet."

In more advanced cases (grades III or IV), this discharge can be strong enough to affect underwear. Some people use pads, others wash multiple times a day. What they all share is the persistent feeling of not being clean or dry – which can deeply affect well-being.

As a result, many subtly change their daily habits: avoiding tight clothing, feeling uncomfortable when sitting, steering clear of long car rides or public restrooms. It's a slow retreat that often goes unnoticed – but can become a significant burden over time.

Why These "Quiet" Symptoms Should Be Taken Seriously

Itching, burning, and moisture may sound minor compared to pain or surgical findings. But anyone who has experienced them knows: they can wear you down – over weeks, months, or even years. Especially when they are misdiagnosed, dismissed, or left untreated.

That's why it's important not to accept vague statements like: "As long as it's not bleeding, it's nothing serious," or "It's just sensitive skin." These symptoms are often early signs of a functional imbalance – and your body is clearly signaling that something isn't quite right.

Conclusion: Small Symptoms, Big Impact

The typical signs of hemorrhoidal disease often begin subtly – with a bit of itching, a slight burning sensation, a barely noticeable feeling of dampness. But these early symptoms deserve real attention. They are not just annoying – they are often the first clues that the body needs support.

Those who take these signs seriously can act early – and in many cases, prevent a minor irritation from becoming a long-term problem.

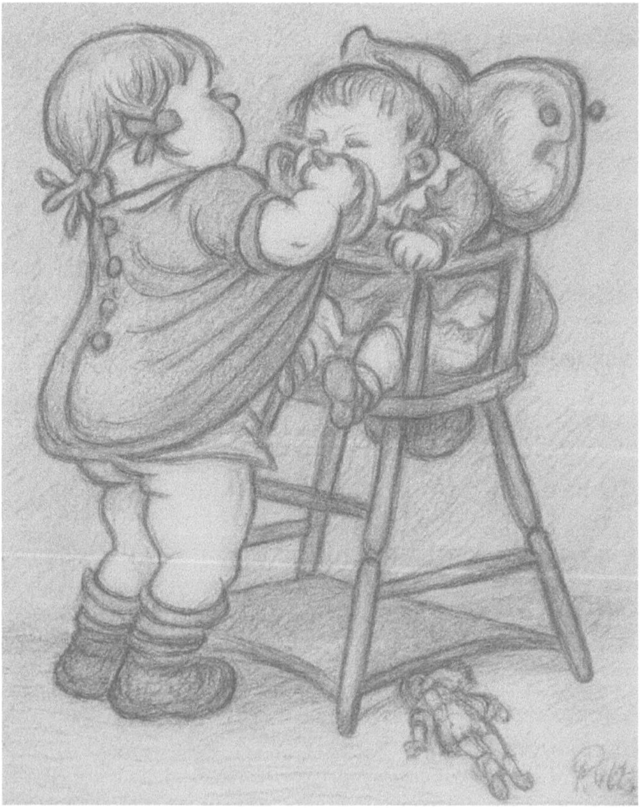

The depiction in the image is definitely not recommended for imitation…

3.2 – Pain During Bowel Movements or Sitting

Not all hemorrhoids are painful. Especially in early stages, hemorrhoidal disease often progresses without significant pain – instead accompanied by more subtle symptoms like itching, moisture, or a feeling of pressure. But as soon as pain occurs during bowel movements or while sitting, many affected individuals realize: a quiet irritation has become a very real problem.

And even though such pain is often downplayed or treated as taboo, it can significantly interfere with daily life.

Pain Is Not Always the Same

Pain in the anal area can manifest in many different ways. Some people feel a sharp or cutting sensation during bowel movements, while others describe a dull pressure afterward. Some report burning irritation that lingers for hours, others describe sudden shooting pain when sitting down – as if pressing on something sore or inflamed.

This makes it complex: there isn't one single type of pain, but many variations – depending on where the issue is located, how far it has progressed, and whether additional irritation, injury, or inflammation is present.

Why Does Pain Occur During Bowel Movements?

The most common trigger is increased mechanical pressure in the rectum. Enlarged hemorrhoids, especially from grade III onward, may prolapse during straining and stretch or pinch sensitive tissue. If there are small tears in the mucosa – for example from hard stool – this can cause burning or even knife-like pain.

Even small tears (anal fissures) that develop from irritation or over-wiping can be extremely painful due to the rich nerve supply and blood flow in the area. Such a tear doesn't just hurt in the moment – the pain can linger for hours, sometimes accompanied by spasms of the sphincter muscle.

In some cases – such as with anal vein thrombosis – significant pain can occur even without a bowel movement, simply due to swelling and internal pressure.

When Sitting Becomes a Challenge

What most people take for granted – sitting in a chair, driving a car, going to the movies – can become a real ordeal for those with advanced hemorrhoids or similar conditions. When the hemorrhoidal tissue has prolapsed or become inflamed, sitting can feel like sitting on a marble or on a sore spot.

Many try to shift their weight, sit at an angle, or avoid prolonged sitting altogether. Some turn to donut cushions, with mixed results. Often, movement helps – walking or standing relieves pressure. But in everyday life, sitting for long periods is often unavoidable – whether at work, while driving, or during travel.

Interestingly, the level of pain does not always reflect the severity of the condition. Some people with only mildly enlarged hemorrhoids experience strong sensitivity – while others with a significant prolapse feel little to no pain.

Painkillers – Relief or Avoidance?

Many people turn to ibuprofen or other pain relievers during acute flare-ups – and in the short term, that's understandable. I myself took high doses of ibuprofen for several days after surgery, simply because the pain was overwhelming.

But in the long run, pain should not just be "pushed away" – its cause needs to be addressed.

When pain becomes a regular occurrence, it's a sign that something in the body is out of balance – whether it's mechanical irritation, inflammation, or a structural tissue change. And in such cases, more than just a pill is needed.

Conclusion: Pain Is a Signal That Deserves Respect

Pain during bowel movements or while sitting is one of the most distressing aspects of hemorrhoidal disease. It may not always be present – but when it is, it demands attention. And rightly so. Pain is not just annoying – it's your body's way of asking for change.

Anyone experiencing pain in this area should not hide it out of shame or try to minimize it. Instead, see it as an invitation to look more closely – and to seek solutions that go beyond quick fixes and offer lasting relief.

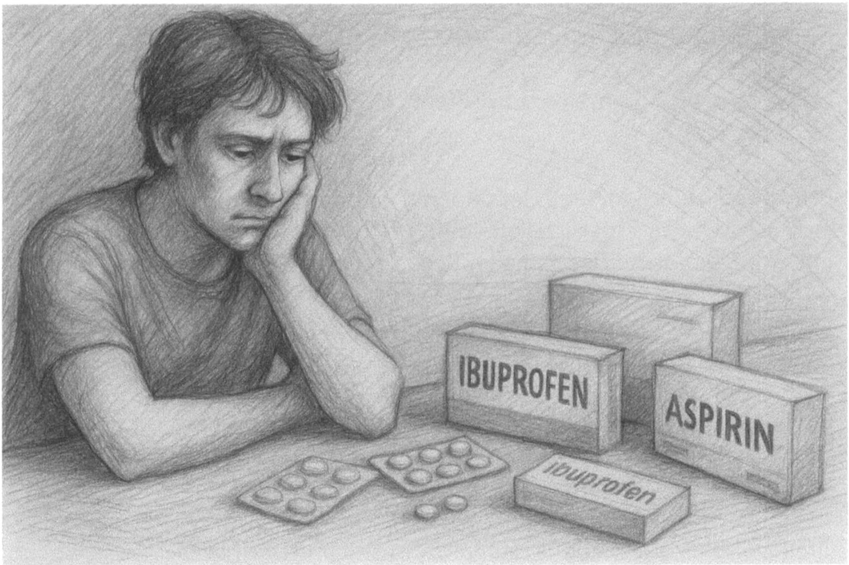

3.3 – Bleeding: When to Take Action

Blood in the stool – even just the thought of it makes many people uneasy. It's a symptom that demands attention immediately. And that's a good thing. Because blood always indicates that a boundary has been breached somewhere in the body – whether due to friction, irritation, inflammation, or a deeper underlying issue.

But not every instance of bleeding signals something dramatic. Especially when related to hemorrhoids, it's important to approach the situation with calm awareness – understanding the difference between what's normal and harmless, and what truly needs medical evaluation.

Bright Red, Dark Red, Mixed – What the Color Reveals

The color of the blood can offer important clues about where the bleeding is coming from:

- **Bright red blood** on the toilet paper or dripping into the bowl usually indicates a fresh, superficial bleeding in the lower rectum – such as from enlarged hemorrhoids or small mucosal tears.
- **Darker blood** or **bloody mucus** mixed with stool may suggest a deeper source of inflammation or bleeding in the upper part of the colon.
- **Black, tar-like stool** (known as melena) is an urgent warning sign – it may point to bleeding in the stomach or small intestine and should be evaluated by a doctor immediately.

With hemorrhoids, the bleeding is typically fresh and bright red, most often after a bowel movement – sometimes visible on the stool, more often on the toilet paper or as drops in the water. It is usually not painful, but can still be alarming, especially if it occurs frequently.

Occasional Bleeding – A Warning, Not an Emergency

Many people with enlarged hemorrhoids experience occasional bleeding – after passing hard stool, sitting for too long, or straining excessively. These episodes are usually brief, stop on their own, and can be reduced with simple changes (such as a softer diet, drinking more fluids, and avoiding straining).

In such cases, it's often enough to observe your habits and make small adjustments. As long as the bleeding is bright red, painless, and not heavy or frequent, there is usually no need for immediate concern.

Recurring or Heavier Bleeding – Take It Seriously

It's a different matter when bleeding:

- Occurs more than once a week,
- Appears in larger, clearly visible amounts,
- Is accompanied by mucus, itching, or burning,
- Persists for several weeks without improvement,
- Or occurs along with other symptoms (e.g. weight loss, fever, changes in bowel habits).

In these cases, a prompt examination by a proctologist is recommended – not because it's automatically dangerous, but to bring clarity. A simple proctoscopy or anoscopy is usually enough to determine the cause. And often, the result is reassuring: it's "just" hemorrhoids – but then you know for sure.

Blood Is a Warning Sign – Even With Hemorrhoids

Even though hemorrhoids are very common and usually harmless, blood should never be considered "normal." It may eventually become part of everyday life for some, but it's still a sign that the tissue is irritated, damaged, or under stress.

Ignoring frequent bleeding increases the risk of chronic irritation, inflammation, and missed opportunities to detect other, more serious causes in time.

One common mistake is to self-treat symptoms – with creams or sitz baths – without a proper diagnosis. Understandable, but risky. Only a specialist can reliably distinguish between hemorrhoids, fissures, polyps, or even a tumor. And even if it's "only" hemorrhoids, early treatment is simpler and more effective.

Conclusion: Early Recognition, Targeted Action

Rectal bleeding is often harmless – but never meaningless. If it happens once, stay observant. If it happens repeatedly, have it checked by a doctor.

The good news: In the vast majority of cases, nothing serious is behind it. But it's reassuring to know that for certain – not just hope so. And those who act early can usually resolve the issue with simple, low-effort measures, before the problem becomes more serious.

Did You Know…?

Sitting on the toilet for extended periods increases pressure on the blood vessels in the anal area and can significantly raise the risk of developing hemorrhoids. Those who regularly linger with their smartphone in hand often extend their time without realizing it – and may be doing more harm than they think.

3.4 – Chronic Discomfort: The Slow Progression

Hemorrhoids rarely start with a bang. There's no day X when everything suddenly changes. No abrupt turning point, no dramatic pain that immediately leads you to a doctor. Instead, it's the quiet signs that gradually creep in over months or even years. And that's exactly what makes them so persistent.

Many sufferers – myself included – don't experience hemorrhoids as a single event, but as a slow development that subtly integrates itself into everyday life. You notice the first symptoms – itching, a bit of burning, an occasional drop of blood – and think nothing of it. Maybe your stool was too hard, maybe you sat too long, maybe the area is just "sensitive." And then life goes on.

But therein lies the risk: we get used to discomforts that aren't actually normal.

From occasional to regular – without noticing it

Chronic hemorrhoids usually develop over years. What begins with occasional itching gradually becomes a daily companion. A single drop of blood turns into a small streak, then becomes a routine occurrence. Later, there's the feeling that "something's off" down there – a slight foreign body sensation, a pressure while sitting, or a vague irritation after using the toilet. Sometimes it feels tight, sometimes itchy, sometimes burning.

And although you sense that something isn't right, you adapt: you wipe differently. You sit for shorter periods. You use soothing ointments. You avoid long trips or change your underwear more often. And eventually, you don't even notice how much your daily life has started to revolve around the problem.

Normalizing the suffering – a silent mistake

What many don't realize: they are no longer living with the issue, but around it. The condition becomes integrated into everyday life – not because it has been understood, but because you've learned how to function despite it.

And this is one of the greatest hurdles in dealing with chronic issues: you lose sight of what "normal" even means.

I myself thought for years that it was just "my body." A bit more sensitive, a little irritated – maybe just genetics. The idea that it might be a treatable, explainable, and possibly curable condition didn't occur to me for a long time. Only when the discomfort became truly severe – almost daily bleeding, the feeling of constant prolapse – did I begin to look at it differently.

The psychological component: silent stress

Chronic conditions are not just physical. They also change how we see ourselves. Many sufferers gradually develop a sense of losing control: "I just can't get a handle on this," or "I just want it to go away." Constant attention to an intimate, often taboo area drains your energy – emotionally, mentally, and often socially.

There's also the uncertainty: What exactly is this? Will I need surgery? Is it dangerous? Can I still exercise? Is this hygienic? These unanswered questions keep circling in your mind – often without ever being discussed with anyone. You Google, you try remedies, you order creams – and hope for improvement without ever gaining true clarity.

Conclusion: Chronic doesn't mean hopeless

Even if hemorrhoids follow a chronic course – that doesn't mean you have to live with them. On the contrary: especially those with long-term discomfort can often achieve more with targeted measures than someone with a one-time acute flare-up. What's important is not to see the body as the enemy, but as a messenger.

Those who listen early can prevent a lot of suffering. And those who have been living with the condition for a while should allow themselves to make a change now – not out of fear, but out of the desire to reconnect with their own well-being.

The path out of the chronic phase often doesn't begin in a waiting room – but with a single sentence you say to yourself:

"I'm taking this seriously now."

Chapter 4: Why So Many People Wait Too Long to Take Action

Those who suffer from hemorrhoids often wait a long time before doing anything about it. Sometimes years pass – sometimes decades. And even though the symptoms keep returning, people suppress them, get used to them, downplay them, or hope they'll just go away on their own. This chapter explores why so many people don't act early – and why that's understandable.

It usually starts with a sense of shame. **Chapter 4.1** – Shame, Insecurity, and Social Taboos looks at how deeply this topic is buried in everyday life. For many people, the bowel is a taboo zone – especially when it comes to blood, burning, or discharge. And yet, millions are affected. Still, those who talk about it feel vulnerable – or so they believe. So they stay silent.

On top of that, many think they know exactly what's going on. **Chapter 4.2** – Misconceptions and Self-Diagnoses describes the typical detours people take: reading something online, hearing something from a friend, or comparing themselves to others – and believing they've got it under control. Harmless symptoms are often overestimated – while serious ones are overlooked. And while one is still figuring it out, the condition becomes chronic.

Even a visit to the family doctor doesn't always help. **Chapter 4.3** – Why Many General Practitioners Can't Provide Help addresses the structural limitations within healthcare. Many GPs are overwhelmed by their daily workload, and examining the rectum is neither popular nor routine. So more weeks and months pass with little or no action – while the problem quietly worsens.

Chapter 4.4 – The First Visit to a Specialist: My Experience finally tells the story of my own journey – the moment I had to admit that things couldn't go on like this. What it was like to visit a clinic specializing in colorectal conditions for the first time. What happened there. And why the experience was both helpful and sobering.

This chapter aims to encourage – while also being honest:

The road to healing often begins late – but it can begin. And it is never too late to take responsibility for your own body.

4.1 – Shame, Insecurity, and Social Taboos

Hemorrhoids are among the most common health conditions worldwide. Yet very few people talk about them openly. Why? Simple: it's embarrassing. Hardly any other part of the body is so deeply associated with shame as the anus. Complaints in this area are often seen as "disgusting," "gross," or simply "inappropriate" – even when they are medically normal and treatable.

When uncertainty takes over

Many affected individuals are initially unsure whether their symptoms are really "something serious." A bit of itching, a mild burning sensation – couldn't that just be from diet? Or from sitting too long? Or from stress? These thoughts are widespread – and often lead to early warning signs being ignored for years. Only when blood appears in the stool or sitting becomes chronically painful does the feeling arise: Now I really need to do something. But by then, the condition has often already progressed to a moderate or advanced stage.

Going to the doctor – a major hurdle for many

No one needs to justify a doctor's visit for back pain or stomach trouble. But talking about anal complaints is extremely difficult for many – even with medical professionals. The idea of being examined "down there" makes many feel exposed or vulnerable. Common thoughts include: "What will the doctor think of me?" or "What if it's something serious?" These insecurities often lead to postponing a medical consultation for far too long.

A culture of silence

To make matters worse, the topic is almost completely absent from public discourse. There is little to no education – neither in schools nor in adult health programs.

Even among friends, it's rarely mentioned seriously – if at all, it shows up only as a joke or figure of speech ("a pain in the ass" – but never truly discussed).

This silence leaves many sufferers feeling alone – even though millions are going through the same thing.

Conclusion: A problem that grows in silence

The combination of shame, uncertainty, and lack of public education causes many people to act too late. Yet early treatment is often simple, gentle, and effective.

Those who are honest with themselves and take the step to seek medical help can spare themselves a lot of suffering – and in some cases even avoid surgery.

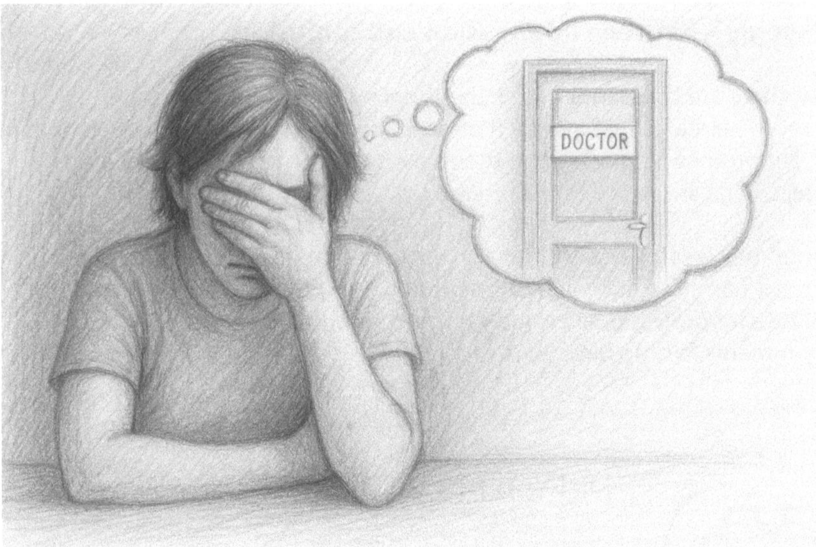

4.2 – Misconceptions and Self-Diagnoses

Many people tend to downplay early symptoms in the anal area.

A bit of itching? Probably just the wrong underwear.

Mild burning? Must be from spicy food.

A drop of blood on the toilet paper?

"Just a small cut, nothing serious."

This kind of self-reassurance is understandable – but often misleading. Hemorrhoidal conditions in particular tend to develop gradually. What starts out as harmless can slowly evolve over months or years into a more serious issue.

Dr. Google – between information and confusion

Today, there are thousands of search results for every symptom online. While this may seem helpful at first glance, it often leads to confusion. Many people search their symptoms and quickly find themselves confronted with terms like anal fissure, colon cancer, or Crohn's disease.

This not only creates anxiety, but also makes it harder to assess the situation: When is it harmless, and when is it serious? Trying to self-diagnose is no substitute for professional evaluation. On the contrary – it often leads to misjudgments in both directions.

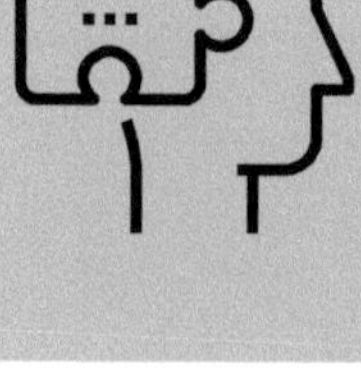

Did You Know…?

Silent suffering can also make you sick.

Feelings of shame often lead people to suppress their symptoms for years – unconsciously increasing their emotional and physical burden.

The limits of self-treatment

Pharmacy shelves are full of ointments, suppositories, and creams for hemorrhoids. Many of these products do relieve symptoms – at least temporarily.

The problem: They treat the symptoms, not the cause.

Those who rely on them may avoid a visit to the doctor in the short term but risk worsening the condition in the background. Especially in the case of Grade III or IV hemorrhoids, topical treatment alone is no longer sufficient. Misjudging the severity and relying solely on self-treatment can waste valuable time.

Mild symptoms – or a warning sign?

Not every symptom in the rectal area is necessarily due to hemorrhoids.

Blood in the stool, for example, can point to a range of other conditions – some of them far more serious. Pain during bowel movements may also have various causes: fissures, fistulas, infections, or even tumors.

Those who rush to diagnose themselves and find false reassurance risk missing or delaying the treatment they truly need.

Conclusion: Knowledge is not a substitute for examination

Misconceptions and self-diagnoses are common – especially when it comes to sensitive issues like anal discomfort. The desire to help oneself is human. But those who experiment for too long on their own not only risk worsening their condition, but also endanger their overall health.

A proper medical evaluation often brings more clarity and peace of mind than hours of Googling ever could.

4.3 – Why Many General Practitioners Can't Really Help

For many people, their general practitioner (GP) is the first point of contact when health issues arise. That's generally a good thing – especially for an initial assessment. But when it comes to hemorrhoidal conditions, GPs often reach their limits quickly. Not because they're incompetent, but simply because their focus lies elsewhere. The field of proctology – dealing with diseases of the rectum – only takes up a small part of medical training. And in everyday practice, the focus is usually on very different issues: high blood pressure, diabetes, infections, psychosomatic complaints.

"You should see a specialist"

Many GPs recognize that something isn't quite right in the anal area – but hesitate to make a definitive diagnosis. Instead, they often give general advice like: "Try a hemorrhoid cream for now," or "It's probably nothing serious." Or they refer the patient directly to a proctologist or gastroenterologist.

For the patient, this can be frustrating: they've already overcome the hurdle of going to the doctor – only to leave without a clear answer. The uncertainty remains.

Physical examination? Often missing

A sensitive topic like anal discomfort requires tact – in both the literal and figurative sense. Many patients secretly hope the doctor will skip the examination. And many GPs, consciously or not, comply with that unspoken wish – out of politeness, time constraints, or simply lack of experience.

Yet a simple visual inspection or brief palpation would often be enough to get an initial picture. That it doesn't happen is one reason why hemorrhoids often go undetected for so long.

Downplaying out of habit

Some GPs tend to dismiss rectal complaints too quickly – partly out of routine, partly due to a lack of specialized knowledge.

Phrases like *"Almost everyone has that at some point" or "Nothing to worry about"* may be well-meaning, but they can have serious consequences.

Not every instance of bleeding is harmless. And not every case of "itching and burning" is a temporary issue. Ignoring such signals for months can allow minor conditions to progress into more serious stages.

GPs matter – but only as a first step

General practitioners are important. They often know their patients for many years, understand their life circumstances, and are usually trusted advisors.

But when it comes to hemorrhoids, the rule is: if you want more than vague statements or standard tips, it's best to consult a specialist early.

Proctologists and colorectal specialists have significantly more experience, better diagnostic tools, and more routine – and can therefore often help more quickly.

What You Can Say or Ask at the Doctor's Office

If you're feeling self-conscious

"This topic is a bit uncomfortable for me, but I've had some anal discomfort for a while – like itching, mild burning, and sometimes blood when I wipe. I'd like to have it checked out."

Why this matters:

Speaking openly helps the doctor take your symptoms seriously. Even if it feels awkward, a clear statement signals that you're ready to act.

If you're unsure

"I read that hemorrhoids have different stages. Can you assess how severe mine might be – or would you recommend I see a specialist?"

Why this matters:

This shows you're informed and engaged. The doctor will see you've taken the topic seriously.

If you're seeking clarity

"I've used ointments a few times, but the symptoms keep coming back. Are there any tests that could help identify the underlying issue?"

Why this matters:

Ointments often just relieve symptoms. Asking about causes leads to a more serious conversation – and more likely a referral to a specialist.

If you want a second opinion

"I feel like the symptoms are getting worse. Could you recommend a good proctologist – or should I find one myself?"

Why this matters:

Sometimes it's helpful to take the next step yourself. Many GPs are even relieved when patients take the initiative.

If you're unsure whether you're in the right place

"I'm not sure if this falls within your area of expertise – but could you take a look, or should I go directly to a specialist?"

Why this matters:

This phrasing is respectful and allows the doctor to respond honestly without feeling confronted.

4.4 – The First Visit to a Specialist: My Experience

At some point, I reached a moment of clarity: things couldn't go on like this. The daily bleeding, the pain, the sensation of a foreign body – it had all become impossible to ignore. A visit to a specialist was long overdue. Through my general practitioner, I received a referral to a gastroenterologist who also specialized in rectal conditions. I didn't know exactly what to expect – but I at least hoped to be taken seriously.

Crowded waiting room, clinical atmosphere

From the first appointment, it became clear I wasn't the only one with these kinds of complaints. The waiting room was completely full. People of all ages, many with tense expressions, some with visible uncertainty on their faces. The atmosphere was cold – professional, almost sterile. No small talk, no music, barely any eye contact. Perhaps I'm projecting in hindsight, but it felt like everyone there wanted to be invisible.

Changing stalls like in a large clinic

When my name was called, I was led down a hallway with several small changing booths – a kind of dressing area you might know from a physical therapy clinic. Four booths in a row, each apparently assigned to one of the adjacent examination rooms. It felt a bit like an assembly line – functional, but not exactly reassuring. I was asked to undress from the waist down and then take a seat in a specialized examination chair.

The first exam – factual, direct, impersonal

The doctor was polite but very matter-of-fact. No small talk, no extended discussion. A quick glance at the screen, a few introductory words – and then the examination.

"This is Grade III to IV," he said after a brief look. He explained that surgery might still be avoidable in my case.

Instead, he recommended treating the hemorrhoids with a method called rubber band ligation – a proven, low-pain approach that could be done over several sessions. I agreed.

Rubber band ligation – unpleasant, but bearable

The first ligation was done on the spot. For those unfamiliar: a small rubber band is placed around the enlarged hemorrhoid, cutting off its blood supply so the tissue dies and falls off after a few days.

It sounds simple – but it doesn't feel that way. On the walk home, I already noticed a strong sensation of pressure. The following days were more than unpleasant. A dull ache, a pulling sensation, sometimes the feeling that something was stuck inside.

Even after the band and tissue had detached, there was residual soreness and discomfort during bowel movements. It was tolerable – but far from harmless.

Interim conclusion: helpful, but not without strain

Although the method made sense medically and probably works well for many patients, I quickly realized it wasn't a sustainable solution for me.

I went through four of these sessions – and felt like it got worse each time. Instead of improving, everything felt more irritated, swollen, and unnatural.

Looking back, that first visit to the specialist was an important step – because it brought clarity. But it was also the moment I realized:

I needed to find my own path, beyond conventional medical treatment alone.

1 2 3 4 5 6 7 8 9 10 11 12 13 14 15 16 A

Part 2: Between Hope and Disillusionment – The Journey Through Conventional Medicine

Chapter 5 – Rubber Band Ligation: A Simple Procedure with Limited Benefits

For many people suffering from persistent hemorrhoid symptoms, rubber band ligation represents the first serious medical intervention. It is considered gentle, quick to perform, and relatively low-risk. These very characteristics make it so popular—and widely used—in proctological practice. This method was also recommended to me early on, as the next logical step after unsuccessful conservative treatment.

This chapter explores what ligation treatment can—and cannot—achieve. I aim to describe how this method works, what it triggers in the body, what expectations are commonly associated with it, and what it actually means in reality when one decides to undergo the procedure.

In the first **section, 5.1**: Mechanism and Course of the Ligation Treatment, I explain the medical rationale behind the procedure: how the rubber band is applied, what happens within the body, and how the process typically unfolds—including the reactions many people experience afterward.

The second **section, 5.2**: Pain, Restlessness, Recurrence – Why It Often Falls Short, highlights the downside of this method. Many patients report ongoing discomfort, sharp pain, or an inner restlessness that is difficult to describe. Recurrences are also common—even after multiple sessions. This chapter explores why, despite working on a technical level, the procedure does not always provide the hoped-for relief.

In the third **section, 5.3**: Personal Experiences with Multiple Sessions, I share my own story: four treatments—some accompanied by significant pain, some with no noticeable effect—and, in the end, my decision to discontinue the ligation therapy altogether. Rather than easing my condition, these sessions increased the sense of distress. Ultimately, this phase became a turning point that led me to consider surgical options.

Chapter 5 is therefore not intended as a medical verdict—but as a personal interim assessment. Rubber band ligation can help. It can bring relief. But it can also lead to disappointment. And it is precisely at that point that the question arises: should one continue to rely on technical procedures—or begin to explore new paths?

5.1 – Mechanism and Course of the Ligation Treatment

Rubber band ligation is a standard medical procedure for treating internal hemorrhoids, particularly in stages II and III. The goal of this method is to selectively cut off the blood supply to the affected tissue by tying it off. As a result, the tissue dies off, detaches on its own after a few days, and the body naturally closes the area with scar tissue. The hope behind this approach: fewer symptoms, less bleeding, and reduced pressure in the anal region.

The Procedure: Quick, but Not Without Preparation

The actual ligation is a relatively brief intervention, often performed on an outpatient basis in a proctologist's office. After a short visual inspection, a special instrument—called a ligator—is used to place a small rubber band around the hemorrhoidal swelling. This step usually takes only a few seconds.

Nevertheless, proper preparation is important. In most cases, the bowel is emptied beforehand, typically with an enema, and it is advisable to avoid strenuous appointments on the day of the procedure. Even though the treatment is considered "simple" from a medical perspective, each body reacts differently—some experience a feeling of pressure, others cramping, and some feel almost nothing at all.

What Happens Afterwards: The Natural Rejection Process

After the procedure, the body begins to react to the tied-off tissue. Within three to seven days, it dies, dries out, and detaches unnoticed during a bowel movement. A small scar forms at the site, which ideally prevents further congestion of hemorrhoidal tissue in that area.

Many patients report a dull pressure or mild discomfort in the first one to two days—especially when sitting or walking. In rare cases, more intense pain may occur, particularly if the rubber band was placed too deep or too close to sensitive tissue. In such situations, it may be helpful to consult a doctor promptly.

Risks and Complications: Rare, but Possible

As with any procedure, rubber band ligation carries risks. In rare cases, heavier bleeding can occur—especially if the detached tissue exposes a sensitive area. Infections, fever, or persistent pain are also possible, though uncommon.

Another risk is of a psychological nature: many patients approach the procedure with high expectations, only to feel disheartened if not all symptoms disappear or if new issues arise. In some cases, the treatment must be repeated several times to achieve a satisfactory outcome.

When Ligation Makes Sense—and When It Doesn't

Rubber band ligation is not a one-size-fits-all solution. It is particularly suited for easily accessible internal hemorrhoids with little or no external involvement. In more advanced cases or when accompanied by skin folds, fissures, or inflammation, the method reaches its limits.

Even so, for many patients, it represents a first attempt—precisely because it is gentle, cost-effective, and relatively low in risk. Some are fortunate and experience genuine relief. Others are less lucky and must then consider further treatment options.

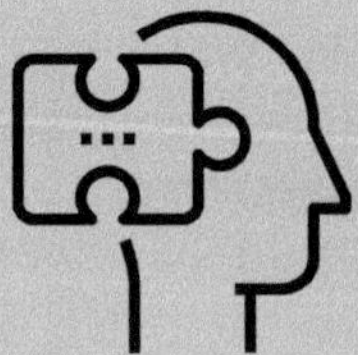

Did You Know…?

Many people affected by hemorrhoids hesitate for years to see a doctor due to shame—and in doing so, accept significant limitations in their daily lives. Yet early stages can often be treated easily, for example with ointments or minimally invasive procedures.

5.2 – Pain, Restlessness, Recurrence – Why It Often Falls Short

For many, rubber band ligation carries a quiet hope: finally some relief, finally a return to feeling at ease in their own body. The idea that the problem can be resolved with just a few simple steps sounds appealing. But reality often paints a different picture. As technically straightforward as the procedure may be—the emotional and physical experience afterward remains complex.

Shortly after the procedure, some patients begin to experience unusual symptoms: a persistent pressure that doesn't subside, pulling pain while walking, and a sense of restlessness in the lower abdomen. Trust in one's own body begins to falter—especially when the symptoms don't improve, but actually worsen.

When the Body Sends a Warning: Pain After Ligation

In theory, ligation is considered to be a low-pain treatment—but in practice, each person experiences it differently. While some feel almost nothing, others react with great sensitivity. It can be especially distressing when the rubber band is positioned unfavorably—too deep, too close to the sensitive mucosa, or near nerve-rich areas.

This can result in persistent pain, which goes far beyond mere pressure. It often feels more like a deep internal irritation that hardly eases—even when lying down. Painkillers offer limited relief, and the question inevitably arises: is this still normal? Or is something wrong?

In some cases, the rubber band is removed early by the doctor—a small procedure, but with a significant psychological impact. What remains is growing doubt: doubt in the body, in the treatment itself, and in the hope for swift improvement.

Inner Restlessness – An Underestimated Companion

Alongside physical pain, inner restlessness can become a major factor. When the feeling that "something isn't right" lingers for days, a state of constant tension can easily develop. Every trip to the bathroom becomes a source of stress, every movement is watched with unease.

Often, it's not the pain itself that makes life difficult, but the constant waiting for things to get worse. The thought, "hopefully this will go well," becomes a silent companion—and can turn into a real psychological burden. Especially when the condition fails to stabilize over several weeks.

Recurrence and Repetition – The Cycle Begins

Another challenge of rubber band ligation is its limited effectiveness. In many cases, one session is not enough. Two, three, or even four appointments may be needed to treat all affected areas. And even then, relapses are not uncommon.

New hemorrhoids can develop, and previous symptoms return—sometimes just a few weeks later. Patients find themselves back at the beginning. Medically monitored, yes—but without the feeling of true progress. The procedure may have eased something—but the problem remains.

Between Hope and Resignation

Those who undergo multiple ligation sessions often lose faith in the prospect of a lasting solution. The appointments become routine, expectations lower, and the willingness to continue fades. It's not uncommon for the thought to arise: "If even this doesn't help—then what?"

This point is crucial. It is often where the search for alternatives begins—for methods that reach deeper, last longer, or are more individually tailored. And this is where personal reflection sets in: how much time, energy, and hope is one still willing to invest in procedures that may be well-established—but are not always sustainable?

5.3 – Personal Experiences with Multiple Sessions

Rubber band ligation is often portrayed as a straightforward procedure that takes only a few minutes and is expected to provide rapid relief. Unfortunately, that was not my experience. I underwent this treatment a total of four times—in the hope that the problem would gradually resolve itself. But the more sessions I went through, the more my doubts grew as to whether this was truly the right path.

Even after the first treatments, I felt a growing sense of discomfort—not only physically, but also mentally. It was not the relief I had hoped for, but rather the feeling that something was "off." With each session, the inflamed area seemed to become more present, as if one were repeatedly treating an open wound. Over time, I became convinced: this type of treatment was not helping me—quite the opposite.

Sharp Pain and the Sensation of a Foreign Body

What affected me most was the specific type of pain I experienced in the days following each ligation. The rubber band didn't just cause pressure; it created a kind of lingering, sharp pain that never fully subsided. It felt as though something was inside me that didn't belong—a constant "foreign element" that my body couldn't ignore.

Even after the band had detached, the sensation of irritation and pain lingered for several days. It wasn't an intense pain, but a constant, underlying discomfort—aggravating, exhausting, and at times draining. Not comparable to major surgery, but ever-present nonetheless. And that wears you down in its own way.

When the Treatment Fails to Deliver

One especially frustrating experience was a session where the ligation simply didn't work. After about three days, the rubber band fell off—but without any tissue. It had likely been placed incorrectly or the hemorrhoidal tissue wasn't sufficiently developed. The result: no effect, no change—just another procedure that cost time, energy, and hope.

Moments like these are difficult to process. You sit there, having endured the pain and come to terms with the procedure—only to find it was all for nothing. No progress, no relief—just the feeling of being stuck in a medical hamster wheel.

The Moment You Decide to Stop

After four sessions, it became clear to me: I was done. It no longer made sense to continue. My symptoms were not improving—if anything, they were getting worse. The feeling of inflammation, of internal pressure and irritation, was becoming more pronounced. It seemed that each new procedure brought more disturbance than help.

And so I made the decision to leave rubber band ligation behind. A few months later, I opted for a different path—the THD operation. A more invasive procedure, with its own challenges, but also with the hope of finally finding a more profound solution.

An Interim Conclusion

Rubber band ligation is certainly a good option for many patients—especially when dealing with clearly defined hemorrhoidal conditions in their early stages. But in my case, it was not the answer. It became more of a transitional phase—a time of searching, of doubt, and of cautious reevaluation: Where does conventional medicine truly help me—and where does it not?

These experiences shaped me. And they taught me how important it is to truly listen to your own body. Not every procedure that makes medical sense brings genuine relief to the individual. Sometimes, the only right step is to walk away—and start thinking anew.

Chapter 6 – The First Operation: THD and Its Pitfalls

After several unsuccessful treatment attempts—including rubber band ligation—I increasingly felt the need for a more lasting solution. The symptoms had begun to dominate my daily life, and my trust in minor interventions had been shaken. So I started to explore surgical options more thoroughly. The range was wide: traditional excision techniques, modern stapler procedures, laser-based approaches—each method had its advantages and disadvantages, its advocates and critics.

In **Section 6.1**, I describe the decision-making process that ultimately led me to the so-called THD method—an operation considered to be minimally invasive, in which the supplying vessels are identified using ultrasound and then ligated. I deliberately chose this method because it was advertised in brochures as particularly low in pain—and in online forums, it seemed to be the most acceptable option among the surgical choices.

The procedure itself took place at a clinic in Duisburg—professionally performed, but within a healthcare system clearly reaching its limits. As a public health insurance patient, I was initially placed in an overcrowded six-bed ward, where I was confronted with conditions that had little to do with genuine medical care.

Section 6.2 focuses on the reality after the operation: the pain, the limitations, the slow and difficult recovery—and the sobering realization that this supposedly "low-pain" procedure turned out to be the most physically taxing operation I had ever experienced. I describe openly how I lived through the days after the surgery, which pain medications I tried, and why daily life during that period became a true test of endurance.

But the real disappointment came later. About three months after the operation, the first signs of a relapse began to appear. At first it was subtle—a slight sense of pressure, a recurring "protrusion"—but over time, it became clear: the problem was returning.

In **Section 6.3**, I recount this recurrence, which unfolded gradually but unmistakably. What began as a small irregularity became a renewed diagnosis—one that eventually looked almost identical to my condition before the surgery. The realization that I had arrived back at square one despite all the effort and pain marked a low point—and at the same time, the beginning of yet another search.

6.1 – The Hope for a Lasting Solution

Taking a bigger step: After several disappointing rubber band ligation sessions and persistent symptoms, I began to long for a more lasting solution. It wasn't a spontaneous decision, but the result of thorough consideration. I read brochures, combed through online forums, spoke with doctors—and quickly realized: the world of hemorrhoid surgeries is complex. There are various methods, sometimes with similar names but different procedures—from traditional cutting techniques to modern stapler methods and minimally invasive approaches using ultrasound or laser.

The THD method—Transanal Hemorrhoidal Dearterialization—eventually appeared to me as the most reasonable path. While the reports I read in online forums were mixed, many sounded at least pragmatic: less pain than traditional surgery, shorter recovery times, and an acceptable risk profile. What particularly appealed to me was the promise of a largely pain-free procedure. The brochure claimed that, due to the targeted ligation of the feeding arteries, hardly any open wounds would result—greatly reducing the risk of pain.

So what exactly is THD?

At its core, the THD method is based on the use of a special proctoscope equipped with a Doppler ultrasound device to locate the arteries supplying blood to the hemorrhoids. These vessels are then ligated with sutures, reducing blood flow so that the tissue shrinks. In many cases, a so-called "mucosal lifting" is performed at the same time—meaning the prolapsed mucosa is lifted back into place and fixed. No removal, no cutting, no stapling—at least according to theory.

Although THD is sometimes described as an alternative to the well-known "stapler methods," there are certainly parallels. Ultimately, these are technical variations of the same principle: reducing blood flow and restoring the tissue to its proper position. The differences lie mainly in how the tissue is fixed—some methods use staples, others use sutures—and in how much tissue is removed or preserved.

The Clinic – Between Professionalism and an Assembly-Line Feeling

I had the procedure done at a clinic in Duisburg. I chose this facility partly because they had experience with the THD method. The process appeared well organized, the staff was friendly, and everything was handled professionally—but it was also clearly a high-volume institution. Even during admission, it was obvious: a large number of patients were being treated here. Everyone got their turn—but the process was tightly scheduled, compressed, efficient.

For me, this meant: very little personal guidance, hardly any room for questions, and a general sense of being a case number rather than a person. This is not meant as a criticism of the staff—they performed their duties with dedication. But the system itself was geared toward high throughput. And that becomes painfully clear when you're going through a vulnerable phase of life.

General Anesthesia and the Moment After

The surgery was performed under general anesthesia. I still remember hoping, just before falling asleep, that this would mark the beginning of a new phase—without pressure, without inflammation, without the constant focus on bowel movements. When I woke up, the hope was still there—but the reality hit immediately: I needed strong painkillers. Even in the recovery room, it was clear that this procedure had not passed without a trace. The anesthesia had worn off—but the pain was present.

Despite being labeled a "gentle" method, my body was on high alert. The affected area felt swollen, raw, and overstimulated. I tried to stay calm—it was, after all, expected that surgery would provoke a reaction. Still, a first doubt crept in, reminiscent of a line by the comedian Loriot: So this is what "low pain" is supposed to mean?

Hospital Reality – In a Six-Bed Room as a Public Health Patient

What I hadn't anticipated—and what remains vivid in my memory—was the situation on the ward itself. As a public health insurance patient, I was placed in a six-bed room. That alone was a challenge: six strangers, different life stories, various illnesses, smells, sounds. But that wasn't the worst part.

One of the other patients was clearly suffering from a severe mental disorder. He seemed confused, disoriented, sometimes speaking incoherently, often unaware of his surroundings. During the day there were already odd scenes—strange noises, spontaneous conversations with himself. But things escalated during the night: around 3:30 a.m., he suddenly got up, turned on the harsh overhead light, got fully dressed, and declared that he had to go to work now. It took a while until a nurse arrived and gently brought him back to bed.

But the situation worsened soon after. He was given a laxative—for medically sound reasons. What might have been manageable in a private room became a disaster in an overcrowded shared one. As could have been expected, less than ten minutes later he lost control. In a state of panic, confusion, and disorientation, he soiled the entire room—including himself. He slipped in his own excrement, appeared helpless, and was barely responsive. It was a moment that was deeply distressing—both physically and emotionally.

I happened to run into the chief physician in the hallway shortly after and calmly but firmly explained what had happened. To my relief, the response was prompt: within half an hour, someone from the staff came and offered me a different room. I was grateful for that.

But the impression remained. It was one of those moments when you realize how thin the healthcare system has become. How little buffer there is. And how helpless you feel when suddenly caught in an exceptional situation—without privacy, without a backup plan.

Did You Know…?

There are supplementary insurance plans that cover single or double rooms during hospital stays. Without additional coverage for treatment by the head physician, these plans often cost only a single-digit monthly premium.

6.2 – The Reality After the Procedure: Pain and Limitations

Immediately after the operation, I was still under the influence of strong painkillers. I no longer recall exactly which medication they gave me—possibly something from the opioid group, certainly something stronger than ibuprofen, perhaps even metamizole. In that state, everything was more or less bearable. The wound was fresh, the body tense—but thanks to the anesthesia, I was able to tolerate the situation at first.

I stayed in the hospital for a total of two nights. The first night I spent in the overcrowded six-bed room, the second at least in a double room. Then I was discharged. Not at my own request—but as part of the clinic's routine process. In principle, a normal procedure. But for me, the consequences were significant.

The Journey Home – A Torture

I had arrived by car—alone. A mistake, as it turned out. The distance from Duisburg to Oldenburg is around 250 kilometers. And even though I had taken painkillers, it was nearly impossible for me to sit normally. I spent the entire drive trying to avoid contact with the seat as much as possible—pressing my back into the seat, tensing my muscles to slightly lift my pelvis, hovering over the cushion, so to speak.

It was pure torture. I remember the feeling vividly: every bump, every uneven stretch of highway sent a jolt directly into the freshly operated area. And despite all hope that the procedure would be a "gentle" method, it became clear to me: this was anything but mild.

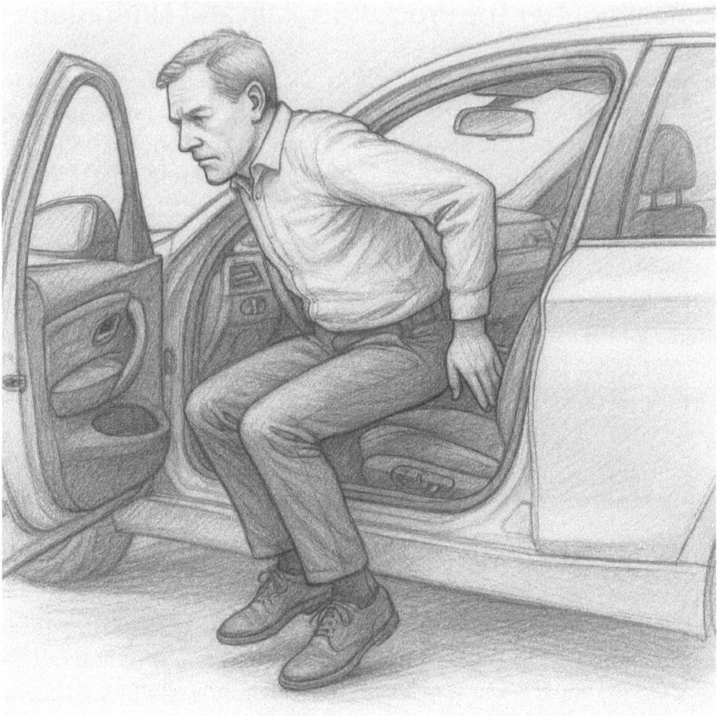

Ten Days Without Sleep – and a Double Dose

In the days that followed at home, things got worse. The pain came in two-hour intervals—like an alarm clock going off at night. Restful sleep was out of the question. I took ibuprofen regularly—first in the recommended dose, then double. Looking back, clearly not a good idea. But at the time, only one thing mattered: keeping the pain under control.

A doctor friend later warned me that this amount of ibuprofen was not without risk—especially for the stomach and kidneys. He brought me a pack of tilidine, a strong opioid-based pain medication. I took one tablet—hoping I could finally sleep through the night. And in fact, the pain felt less intrusive, more distant. But it wasn't completely gone.

What bothered me even more was the aftereffect the next morning. I felt foggy, tired, unfocused—as if someone had stolen half the day from me. A hangover unlike any I had ever experienced with other medications. It quickly became clear: this was not a viable solution. I returned to ibuprofen—with a guilty conscience, but with a clear effect.

Slow Improvement – But Not an Easy Path

After about ten days, things started to improve. Not suddenly, but gradually. Sleep slowly returned, pain peaks became less frequent. Only after three to four weeks was I able to say that I could move more or less pain-free again—even if everything still felt fragile.

In retrospect, it was by far the most painful medical procedure I have ever experienced. And that, despite the fact that THD is considered "minimally invasive." Perhaps I'm particularly sensitive to pain. Perhaps the procedure was more complicated than I had been told. Perhaps it was simply bad luck. But one thing is certain: the reality after the operation was far more difficult than I had expected.

Caution with Opioid-Based Painkillers

After surgical procedures like a THD operation, strong painkillers are sometimes prescribed – including opioid-based medications. While they can offer short-term relief, they come with significant risks: opioids suppress the central nervous system, often cause fatigue or drowsiness, and frequently lead to constipation – which can be especially problematic in the sensitive rectal area.

There's also the risk of dependency or tolerance if used over an extended period. That's why caution is essential when it comes to opioids. If you're experiencing severe pain after surgery, it's advisable to work with your doctor to explore well-tolerated alternatives – and to consider non-pharmaceutical approaches like cooling, relaxation, or gentle movement.

6.3 – The Relapse After Three Months

The weeks following the surgery were marked by pain—but also by hope. I wanted to believe that it had all been worth it. That this procedure, as difficult as it had been, had brought lasting change. And at first, it seemed that way. The symptoms subsided, the pressure sensation was gone, and daily life became a bit easier again.

But after about three months, something began to shift. At first very subtly: a slight pulling sensation during bowel movements, a vague feeling that "something is there again." I tried to ignore it—perhaps it was just my imagination, or a temporary irritation. But the feeling didn't go away. And over time, it became more noticeable.

Relapse Triggered by Small Things – Alcohol, Spice, Everyday Life

I especially noticed it after having a beer or two. Alcohol—even in small amounts—seemed to have an immediate effect. Wheat beer was particularly problematic. The next day, I would feel a change in the anal area: an uncomfortable sense of pressure, the familiar "protrusion" that I had known all too well from before.

Spicy foods—which I largely avoided anyway—also had an immediate effect whenever I made an exception. Anything even slightly irritating seemed to reactivate the sensitive tissue. It was as if the surgery had never taken place. The old irritation mechanism was back—barely three months after the procedure.

From a Pea to a Cherry – Gradual Deterioration

What began as a small lump—about the size of a pea—gradually grew more pronounced. Over the course of a year, it developed once again into a protrusion that, in size, shape, and discomfort, was barely distinguishable from the condition before the operation. Once again, the sensation of a foreign body. Once again, the tiresome need to push it back in. Once again, that sense of uncertainty with movement and everyday activity.

In the end, the diagnosis—objectively speaking—had returned to stage three or even four. After what was considered a "modern" operation, after weeks of pain and limitations, after months of hope, I found myself, emotionally, back at square one.

Follow-Up Visit with a New Surprise

I also recall the follow-up examination about a month after the surgery. At that time, everything still looked fine externally—the surgeon confirmed that the healing process appeared to be progressing well. But during that appointment, something completely unexpected came up: I was told that a fistula had been discovered in a different area during the operation, and that it really should be treated.

I was surprised—because I had never experienced any symptoms in that area. No itching, no discharge, no pain. And in the ten years since, nothing has changed. For me, the remark was more confusing than helpful. It highlighted again how the clinical picture can sometimes differ greatly from what the patient actually experiences—and how easily a secondary diagnosis can become a new issue if you don't stay alert.

Disappointment – But Also Clarity

This experience was crushing. It wasn't just a setback—it was an emotional blow. I had invested so much: time, courage, pain, trust. And now everything had returned. Not with the same intensity—but clear enough to know: this was not the lasting solution I had hoped for.

And yet, this relapse also brought something else: a new sense of clarity. I began to understand more clearly how my body responded—what irritated it, what overwhelmed it. And I knew: if I didn't want to fall into the same cycle again, I would have to find another way—one beyond technology, beyond routine interventions.

Chapter 7 – The Second Operation: Laser Treatment as an Alternative

After the relapse a few months following my first surgery, it became clear to me that I would have to take further action. The symptoms had returned—albeit more gradually—and I didn't want to wait until things worsened again to the level they had been before. But unlike the first operation, this time I approached the situation with a certain emotional distance. I had learned that not everything labeled as "modern" automatically leads to lasting results. Still, I chose to undergo another procedure—hoping that this time, things might turn out differently.

In **Section 7.1**, I discuss the technical differences compared to the THD method. The laser treatment (LHP) does not involve sutures or tissue fixation, but instead works with targeted thermal energy. The affected hemorrhoidal tissue is shrunk from the inside and broken down by the body itself—without external incisions and without visible wounds. To me, this method sounded gentler, more precise, and less invasive—and I was willing to give it a chance.

In fact, the initial phase after the procedure was very positive. In **Section 7.2**, I describe the advantages I experienced in the immediate aftercare following the laser treatment. I was able to sit normally again the very same day, didn't need any pain medication, and for the first time in a long while, I was able to sleep through the night. It almost felt like this had finally been the right step. No side effects, no dramatic reactions—just peace.

But even this hope didn't last. In **Section 7.3**, I explain why this procedure, too, failed to provide a lasting solution. Around three months after the operation, the symptoms gradually returned—subtly, but unmistakably. Once again, my body reacted to the smallest triggers, a new lump began to form, and the sense returned that the core problem had not truly changed. It was only at this point that I began to ask myself whether hemorrhoids might not be a condition in themselves—but rather a symptom of something deeper. A question that fundamentally shifts the focus toward root causes, underlying patterns, and one's personal lifestyle.

7.1 – Technical Differences from the THD Method

After the relapse, one thing was clear to me: I had to try something different. While the first operation had brought short-term relief, the results had not lasted. I was once again experiencing pain, limitations—and a clearly noticeable lump. So I began researching again. This time, my attention was drawn to a procedure known as laser treatment for hemorrhoids, often abbreviated as LHP—Laser Hemorrhoidoplasty.

Compared to the THD method, the procedure sounded technically different—more refined, more precise, more modern. While THD involves locating the feeding arteries with the help of a Doppler sensor and then tying them off with sutures, the laser procedure aims to cauterize the hemorrhoidal tissue itself through targeted energy. The surrounding tissue is largely left untouched—there are no open wounds, no visible incisions, and no external sutures. The treated tissue is meant to be broken down by the body gradually—from the inside out.

Less Mechanical, More Thermal

While THD brings about change by mechanically interrupting blood flow—tying off vessels—the laser treatment works through the application of targeted heat. A thin laser fiber is inserted into the hemorrhoidal cushion. Laser pulses generate heat, causing the vascular tissue to shrink and triggering a controlled inflammatory response. The tissue doesn't die off immediately, but is gradually broken down by the body over days and weeks and replaced with scar tissue.

This approach has several advantages: no open wounds in the anal area, a reduced risk of infection, and—according to providers—significantly less pain during the healing phase. Unlike THD, there is no lifting or suturing of tissue, only a purely thermal effect. No Doppler, no sutures, no foreign material left inside the body. Just targeted laser energy.

Different Equipment, Different Risks

From a technical standpoint, the laser procedure is a completely different concept than the THD operation. Instead of tying off vessels and repositioning mucosa, this method destroys the tissue from within. It requires specialized equipment: a laser diode, fiber-optic system, and control unit. The procedure demands a certain level of experience—not every clinic offers it, and not every physician is equally proficient in it.

Another difference lies in visual control. While THD is performed with direct visual access via a proctoscope, the laser probe is used in a more "blind" fashion—the precise positioning is based on the surgeon's anatomical knowledge and standardized zones within the hemorrhoidal region. This is not necessarily a disadvantage, but it does require a high level of trust in the practitioner's expertise.

Minimally Invasive—But Not Without Impact

The term minimally invasive is also often used in reference to laser treatment. And indeed, from the outside, the procedure appears very mild: no bandages, no visible wounds, no sutures. Still, it is a procedure on a highly sensitive part of the body. The body reacts—with swelling, signs of inflammation, and tension. But the idea is clear: the gentler the method, the faster the healing and the lower the risk of recurrence.

To me, it sounded like a promising alternative—especially after my experience with THD, which, although technically advanced, turned out to be unexpectedly burdensome. I was seeking a solution that would involve less mechanical interference, no internal sutures—and would give my body more space to heal on its own.

7.2 – Advantages in Aftercare

Already on the day of the operation, I realized: this treatment was different. Not just technically, but especially in terms of how it felt afterward. Whereas I had struggled with severe pain for days after the THD procedure, this time the sensation was noticeably milder from the very beginning. No sharp wound pain, no paralyzing feeling of pressure—just a light, dull sensation in the background. Nothing that seriously burdened me.

I was able to sit down immediately after the procedure. And compared to the first surgery, that was almost a key experience for me. No tense posture in the car, no hovering above the chair, no constant effort to avoid movement. It felt as though my body had truly been spared this time—despite the intervention.

No Painkillers – And No Waking Up at Night

The days that followed remained calm. I didn't need any pain medication. No ibuprofen, no tilidine, no nighttime alarms from my nervous system. For the first time after a hemorrhoid procedure, I was actually able to sleep through the night—something that would have been unthinkable after the first surgery. My body seemed to respond well to the laser treatment. No fever, no postoperative bleeding, no serious irritation.

This smooth recovery process was an enormous relief. Especially in contrast to the pain-filled period after the THD, this was a completely different experience. I didn't feel fully healthy—but I felt stable. And at that moment, that meant a great deal.

A First Ray of Hope – Without False Euphoria

Of course, I was aware that the immediate aftermath of a procedure doesn't necessarily say much about the long-term outcome. But the calm of those first few days had an effect on me. No drama, no sense of emergency, no internal state of alarm. I could focus on healing without having to fight against constant pain. For the first time in a long while, it felt like a treatment that truly helped my body—one that didn't overwhelm it, but supported it. And even though I remained cautious not to hope for too much too soon, one thing was clear: postoperative care for hemorrhoids had never felt this manageable before.

7.3 – Why This Procedure, Too, Was Not a Lasting Solution

The first few weeks after the laser treatment felt almost like a small fresh start. I was pain-free, able to sit, sleep, and move without constantly being reminded of my body. No medication, no restrictions in daily life, no constant checking or monitoring. It felt as if my body had finally received what it truly needed.

But once again, the phase of calm was only temporary.

The Relapse – Again, After About Three Months

After around three months, a familiar sensation slowly began to return. At first, it only appeared occasionally, triggered by specific situations—like after drinking one or two beers. It was particularly noticeable with wheat beer or when I accidentally ate something spicy. The anal area responded immediately: with a sense of pressure, a slight prolapse, a familiar "pushing out" feeling I knew all too well.

I monitored it closely. At first, I didn't want to believe it—maybe it was just a minor irritation. But after a few weeks, it became clear: the pattern was repeating itself. What had started as a small irregularity once again became a noticeable lump. A node, initially the size of a pea, gradually grew until it was almost indistinguishable from how things had been before the second operation.

It was the second relapse—despite two modern procedures that were both considered gentle and minimally invasive.

When Nothing Changes, Despite Changing Everything

That moment was sobering. I had gone through two procedures—both with the intention of finally solving the problem for good. Both times, I had hoped it would work. Both times, I had followed medical advice, done everything by the book. And yet, I found myself back in the same place.

This inevitably led to a new question—and a shift in perspective.

A Change in Perspective Begins

Slowly, but with growing clarity, a thought began to take shape: maybe the root cause of the hemorrhoids wasn't located in the anal area at all. Maybe they were just a symptom—a sign of something deeper. A misalignment. An inner tension. An inflammation not caused locally, but supported by systemic factors. Something rooted in gut health, digestion, the nervous system—or even lifestyle itself.

Because if two technically very different procedures—one involving sutures, the other using laser—led to the same result, then perhaps the issue didn't lie in the technique. But in the approach itself.

This realization was not pleasant—but it was necessary. It marked the beginning of a new kind of thinking—away from purely technical solutions and toward a deeper understanding of my body and the signals it was sending.

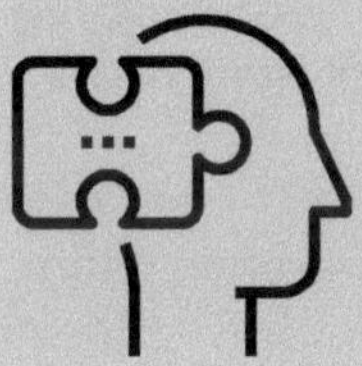

Did You Know...?

A low-fiber diet is one of the main factors contributing to the development of hemorrhoids. People who eat too little fruit, vegetables, and whole grains often experience hard stools—which, over time, puts excessive strain on the blood vessels in the anal area during bowel movements.

Chapter 8 – What Conventional Medicine Can Do – and What It Can't

After two surgeries and numerous treatments, it became increasingly clear to me: conventional medicine has its strengths—but also its limits. It can repair many things, but it rarely truly heals. Especially when it comes to chronic conditions, the standardized thinking in terms of symptoms, procedures, and guidelines eventually reaches its structural boundaries. What initially seemed like a clear medical pathway began to feel more like a roundabout—always leading back to the starting point.

In **Section 8.1**, I begin by addressing the core issue: the focus on symptoms rather than root causes. Medicine treats what it can see—nodules, swelling, bleeding—but often fails to ask why these symptoms developed in the first place. A holistic view of the person—their posture, lifestyle, and internal tension—usually remains in the background.

Section 8.2 explores the high status of technical procedures, which are now applied almost reflexively. Surgeries are considered a standard part of treatment, and minimally invasive methods are presented as solutions. But technology alone cannot replace a real understanding of deeper connections—let alone of the patient's actual lived experience.

In **Section 8.3**, I look at the question of why chronic conditions so often return. Because even if a procedure is deemed a formal success, the problem frequently comes back months or years later. Why? Because the true causes have not been addressed—or because the body has learned to express stress or imbalance through these symptoms. Without systemic change, the effects remain short-lived.

And in **Section 8.4**, I describe my decision to seek a new path. I chose not to undergo any further surgery—and instead began to dig deeper: into my diet, my posture, my inner balance. And eventually, many years later, I stumbled upon what may have been the root cause—a previously undiagnosed case of CMD (craniomandibular dysfunction) that had led to a misalignment of the pelvis. This may well have laid the foundation for my recurring symptoms.

Thus, Chapter 8 marks a turning point: away from medical dependency—toward self-responsibility and a deeper understanding of the body.

8.1 – Symptom-Focused Treatment Instead of Root Cause Exploration

Conventional medicine has countless tools at its disposal. It can cut, cauterize, ligate, fix, and remove. It can relieve pain with medication, reduce inflammation, and stabilize vital functions. It can make many things visible—through ultrasound, endoscopy, or CT scans. In acute cases, this is a blessing—and often life-saving.

But when it comes to treating chronic conditions—especially illnesses like hemorrhoids—a fundamental issue becomes apparent: conventional medicine is trained to identify and treat symptoms. It follows a clear, practical logic: if something protrudes, it is pushed back or removed. If something bleeds, it is cauterized. If something causes discomfort, it is cut away.

What it often fails to ask is: Why did this happen in the first place? What threw the body out of balance? And why does the problem keep returning despite treatment?

Focused on What's Visible—Not on the Whole

In my conversations with doctors—whether general practitioners, proctologists, or surgeons—I repeatedly noticed: the question of the underlying cause was often not raised at all. Or it was quickly dismissed with statements like: "That's just something many people get," or "It's due to your connective tissue," or "You sit too much." And sometimes: "There's not much we can do—just treat it when it gets worse."

At first, these answers sound pragmatic—but they fall short. They stay on the surface. They treat the body like a mechanical system that breaks down in parts—but show little interest in what throws the entire system off balance.

Symptoms are seen as isolated malfunctions that can be fixed independently. The idea that a physical symptom might also be an expression of internal processes, systemic tension, or misdirected regeneration plays little to no role in standard treatment models.

The Patient Becomes the Problem Area

This became particularly clear to me during the course of my two operations. Both procedures were technically precise, both were carried out professionally—but both focused solely on the site of the symptom. The rest of my body—my digestion, my nervous system, my lifestyle, my inner tension—was not considered relevant.

I was not seen as a whole system, but rather as a localized problem area. And that's where the intervention took place. It's an approach aimed at quick results—but rarely equipped for long-term stability. Because the body reacts for a reason. If you only eliminate the reaction without understanding the cause, it will eventually return.

The Difference Between Healing and Repair

Conventional medicine is excellent at repairing. But healing is something else. Healing means restoring balance that has been lost. It means listening, understanding, and going deeper. That's not always possible in a busy hospital or under the time constraints of an insurance-based clinic—and it's not something that should be blamed on individual doctors. But as a patient, you feel these limits very clearly.

The more often I was confronted with the issue, the clearer it became: if I truly wanted to be free of this problem, focusing on the symptom alone wouldn't be enough. I needed to understand why my body kept responding in the same way—despite all the procedures. And that was the point at which my path began to shift—away from relying solely on conventional medicine, and toward something broader that could go deeper.

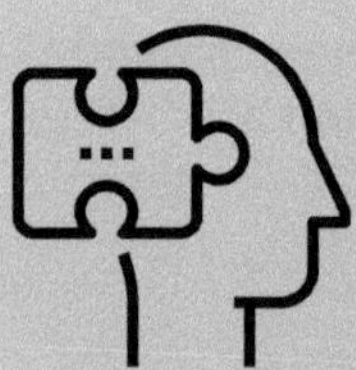

Did You Know…?

Sitting on the toilet for extended periods increases pressure on the blood vessels in the anal area and significantly raises the risk of developing hemorrhoids. Those who regularly "linger" with a smartphone in hand often extend their time on the toilet—and unknowingly harm themselves. It is recommended to limit each visit to the toilet to a maximum of five minutes.

8.2 – The High Value Placed on Technical Procedures

In modern medicine, technology occupies a central role. Surgical techniques are becoming ever more precise, equipment increasingly powerful, and procedures more minimally invasive. Consultations are accompanied by diagrams, proctoscopes come equipped with lights and cameras, and even the smallest blood vessels can be located with targeted ultrasound. It sounds advanced—and in many ways, it truly is.

But this focus on the technical changes the perspective. The more procedures are available, the more attention shifts toward what can be done—not necessarily what needs to be done. Today, there is a technical solution for almost every complaint. And along with that often comes the mindset: if we can do something, then we should.

In my case, this meant two surgeries. One using suture-based THD, and one with laser (LHP). Both modern, both precise, both professionally executed. But neither brought lasting success.

The Allure of What Is Technically Possible

Especially in proctology—the field dealing with rectal and anal disorders—a wide range of procedures has emerged. There are stapler operations, ligation techniques, laser treatments, sclerotherapy, infrared therapy, cryotherapy. Each of these methods has its own advantages, indications, and technical refinements. And all are marketed with the promise of being as effective and painless as possible.

The issue is not the technology itself—but the way it becomes an end in itself. When everything revolves around the procedure, it's easy to lose sight of the person behind it. Their lifestyle. Their diet. Their emotional state. Their everyday reality. At that point, the technology doesn't just replace the illness—it also replaces the thinking in deeper connections.

The System Works—But Does It Heal?

When preparing for surgery, patients are usually given a technical rundown: what will happen in the body, how the device works, how long the procedure takes. But rarely is there discussion about what the body actually needs afterward in order to truly recover. The technology "does its job"—but whether the body makes something good out of it is another matter entirely.

In my case, both procedures worked exactly as they were designed to. The vessels were tied off. The tissue was cauterized. The interventions were effective—but my body still responded with a relapse. Not because the technology failed, but because it wasn't enough.

The Silent Pressure of Standardization

In a highly technologized medical system, there is structural pressure toward standardization. The clearer and more billable a procedure is, the more often it gets used. From an economic perspective, this makes sense—but it also means that individual factors are often overlooked.

Patients who don't respond according to the expected pattern are quickly labeled as "complicated" or "beyond treatment." Yet what they might need most is for someone to shift their focus away from the procedure—and back to the person.

Technology Can Help—But It Can't Replace

I'm not against modern medicine. On the contrary: I'm deeply grateful for many of its advancements. But I've also come to see that technology alone is not enough. It can ease symptoms, treat tissue, simplify procedures—but it cannot replace true, holistic healing. That requires more. A different perspective. A different kind of listening. And sometimes, the courage to explore new paths.

8.3 – Why Chronic Conditions Often Return

Modern medicine is highly effective at treating symptoms. Pain can be relieved, swelling reduced, and problematic tissue removed. This offers patients short-term relief—and often, renewed hope. You feel capable again. You think: Now it's over.

But what happens if the underlying cause remains?

This is the core issue with many chronic conditions. The body uses a symptom to signal that something is out of balance. If the symptom is treated—without identifying the root cause—it may disappear temporarily. But it will very likely return. Because the underlying conditions haven't changed.

The Body Doesn't Forget

In my case, this became especially clear. Both operations—THD and the laser procedure—successfully removed the visible problem for a time. And yet, a few months later, the symptoms returned. Not because there was a technical failure—but because my body remained under a level of strain that surgery alone could not resolve.

The body is not unintelligent. It doesn't repeat symptoms "out of habit." It does so because it needs them—to regulate or compensate for something. When a symptom reappears after treatment, it's not random—it's a sign that the body still perceives the disturbance and continues to respond accordingly.

Lack of Relief, Lack of Change

Chronic conditions often come back because a patient's daily life hasn't changed. Stress, lack of movement, poor nutrition, inner tension, imbalanced physical strain, insufficient recovery—all of this frequently stays the same. And if the body has learned to respond to such persistent stress through specific symptoms, it is highly likely to use the same pathways again.

Surgical procedures can interrupt symptoms—they can act locally—but they don't "unlearn" the body's established patterns. Nor do they automatically resolve systemic causes. That's why so many people with chronic conditions end up back where they started, despite having undergone treatment.

The Recurrence Is Part of the Pattern

For many patients—including myself—it was initially hard to accept that a relapse is not necessarily a medical failure, but often part of a larger pattern. The body doesn't speak up to work against us—it speaks up to be heard. When symptoms return, it's saying: I understand what you fixed mechanically—but that's not enough for me.

This realization is uncomfortable—but it changes the perspective. It moves you away from the passive expectation that a doctor will simply "fix it," and toward a more active, self-responsible stance. You begin to ask: What can I change so that my body no longer has to sound the alarm?

The Key Often Lies Beyond the Symptom

The return of a symptom is often a sign of something deeper: a lack of balance, ongoing overload, or a life situation that has been ignored. Those who recognize these patterns—and begin to change them—have a much better chance of breaking the cycle.

For me, that was the moment I stopped viewing hemorrhoids as just a symptom—and started listening to the message behind them. A decision that changed a great deal.

8.4 – The Decision to Seek a New Path

After two surgeries, countless treatment sessions, and innumerable hours of hoping, one thing had become clear to me: I would not undergo another operation. Not because I fundamentally reject conventional medicine—but because I had realized that it could not answer the central question in my case: Why does this keep coming back?

I had gone through two completely different surgical methods. Both were professionally performed. Both led to short-term improvement. And both ended in the same problem resurfacing just a few months later. It felt like closing a window—only for the wind to find its way back in through another crack.

I wanted to understand what was behind these symptoms. Not just from a technical standpoint, but structurally. And so, I began to search for new paths.

Trial and Error – The Long Journey Through Recommendations and Remedies

In the time that followed, I tried many things. I read forums, personal accounts, and professional articles. I tested nutritional supplements, tried different probiotics, herbal remedies, medicinal plants, and gut detox protocols. I significantly increased my fiber intake, took psyllium husks regularly, and paid attention to proper hydration. Sometimes something helped—sometimes not.

A few remedies improved stool consistency or reduced the sensation of pressure in the short term. Others caused bloating or only made things more complicated. And although some measures felt pleasant, I realized: I was still operating at the symptom level. I was trying to soften the effects—but I still didn't know the root cause.

A Shift in Perspective: From the Anus to the Atlas

What I didn't yet know at the time was that the crucial realization would come many years later—and that it had nothing to do with the rectum, but with the jaw.

Only through a completely unrelated medical context did I discover that I had been living for many years with an **undiagnosed case of craniomandibular dysfunction (CMD)**—a misalignment of the jaw joint that can affect the entire body. In my case, it apparently led to a slight but permanent tilt in the pelvis—which may in turn have caused chronic strain in the lower pelvic region. And possibly contributed to the recurring hemorrhoids.

Whether this is the full truth or just part of it, I cannot say with absolute certainty. But many signs point in that direction—and for the first time, I felt that I was no longer working on the symptom, but on the pattern behind it.

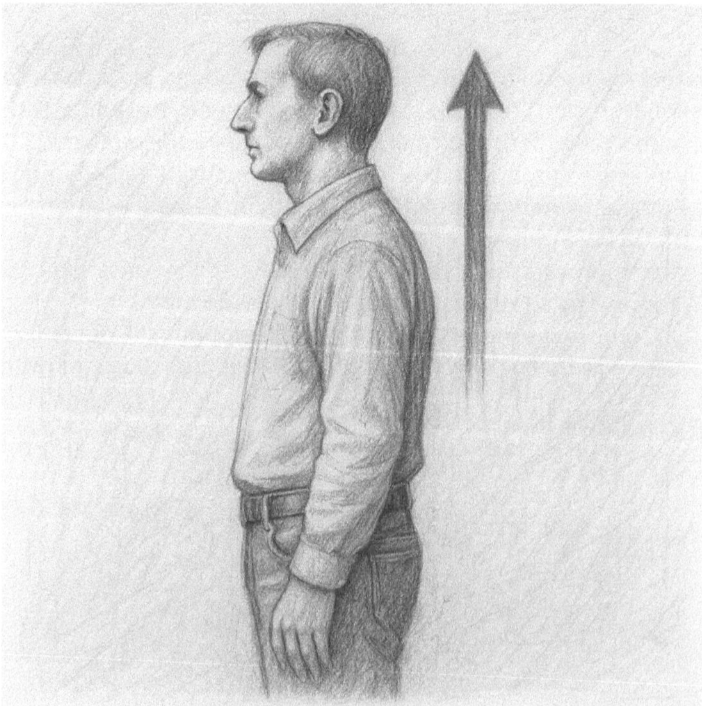

The Beginning of a Different Path

Looking back, the decision not to allow a third operation marked a turning point. I had accepted that the body does not wait for linear solutions—it waits for understanding. And I had begun to see myself as a whole—not just as a "patient with an anal problem," but as a person with posture, tension, habits, and imbalances.

The path was not easy. It didn't bring immediate success. But it was the first step in a new direction. A direction where healing does not begin with technology—but with the courage to look closely. Even in places you least expect it.

Did You Know…?

A pelvic misalignment or poor posture can alter the pressure on the rectum—potentially affecting hemorrhoids and other related conditions. In cases of grade III or IV hemorrhoids, the pelvic floor may also play a role. Targeted pelvic floor weakness is often a contributing factor—and is frequently treatable.

Part 3: A Holistic Perspective – What Might Really Be Behind Hemorrhoids

Chapter 9 – Physical Connections: The Role of Posture and Tension

After many medical treatments and recurring setbacks, I gradually began to shift my perspective. I started asking myself questions that no one had ever asked me before: What does my body actually do all day? How do I stand, how do I sit, how do I breathe? Where do I unconsciously hold tension? Where do I cling to things that should actually be released? And suddenly, areas came into focus that had never seemed relevant before – like my pelvis, my jaw, and my posture in everyday life.

Chapter 9.1 addresses postural imbalances, muscular tension, and pelvic strain. I describe how years of subtle misalignments can negatively impact pressure distribution within the body – potentially leading to chronic irritation in the rectal area. The body compensates for a long time, but eventually the effects begin to surface. Often not where you'd expect them.

A key element in this is the pelvic floor, which I explore in **Chapter 9.2**. It's the silent center where stability, posture, and internal pressure balance converge. In my case, it had been unconsciously overstrained for years – not through strength, but through constant tension. Only when I learned to perceive and relax this area consciously did real change begin.

Chapter 9.3 brought an unexpected twist: jaw misalignments (TMJ dysfunction) and their effect on overall body posture. Long overlooked, it turned out that my jaw joint may have been the root cause of my pelvic tilt – and indirectly of my hemorrhoid issues. At first glance, the connection seems unusual, but within the body's structural system, it makes surprising sense.

Finally, in **Chapter 9.4**, I share my personal observations during the course of my TMJ treatment. Over a period of one to two years – supported by a custom bite splint and complementary therapies – the symptoms gradually began to improve. No surgery, no dramatic intervention – just a slow return to healthier structural balance.

For me, it was a turning point.

9.1 – Postural Imbalances, Tension, and Pelvic Strain

The human body is a finely tuned system of posture, movement, tension, and balance. As long as this interplay functions smoothly, we hardly notice it. Only when individual elements fall out of alignment do symptoms begin to appear – often far from their actual point of origin.

That was likely the case for me. Over many years, I had unconsciously developed postural and muscular tension patterns that led to chronic strain in the pelvic area – potentially laying the foundation for my recurring hemorrhoids. The idea that a postural imbalance or muscular tension could affect venous drainage in the pelvis might sound far-fetched at first – but anatomically, it's more than plausible.

The invisible burden in the pelvic area

Tension tends to accumulate especially quickly in the lower back and pelvic region – whether from prolonged sitting, repetitive movement patterns, weak musculature, or simply years of "incorrect" standing. When the body is no longer evenly loaded, it starts to compensate: some muscles tense up, others weaken, and the pelvis tilts slightly forward or backward.

This subtle shift often goes unnoticed – but it alters the pressure dynamics in the abdominal and pelvic regions. That has a direct impact on the pelvic floor, on venous return, and on the mechanical load placed on the rectum. In my case, I suspect this shift caused a silent yet persistent irritation over the years – which eventually manifested as hemorrhoids.

The body compensates – until it no longer can

Postural issues rarely appear overnight. They result from habits, life circumstances, and years of repetition. The body is remarkably adaptive – but every compensation comes at a cost.

If the hips are slightly misaligned, the spine must counterbalance. If the shoulders slump forward, the neck tightens. And if the pelvis is no longer centered, that pressure also affects the anal canal and surrounding structures.

What's more, those who carry subconscious tension – due to stress or emotional strain – often reinforce these patterns. The result is chronically elevated muscle tone, which not only restricts mobility but also impairs circulation. And impaired circulation plays a central role in the development of hemorrhoids.

The path to awareness – in hindsight

At the time, I wasn't aware of any of these connections. I thought in terms of symptoms, local irritation, and surgical interventions. Only through engaging more deeply with my own body – through observation, bodywork, and eventually a TMJ (CMD) diagnosis – did I begin to realize that the root of my problem likely wasn't "at the exit," but much higher up: in my postural system, in muscular chains, in long-standing patterns.

This insight didn't come from a single lightbulb moment, but from years of observation and countless small puzzle pieces falling into place. But it fundamentally changed how I view the body. Today, I no longer see hemorrhoids as a purely local issue – but rather as a possible consequence of a chronically imbalanced system of tension and strain that begins much earlier than we typically assume.

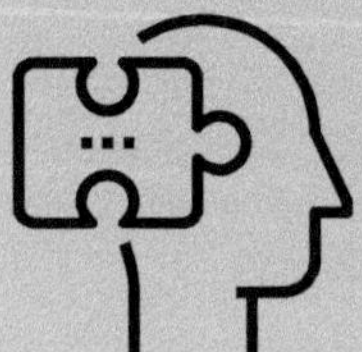

Did You Know...?

Hemorrhoids can be mistaken for irritable bowel syndrome—both conditions can cause pain, a feeling of pressure, and irregular bowel movements. A precise diagnosis is therefore essential.

9.2 – The Importance of the Pelvic Floor

The pelvic floor is one of the most underestimated muscle regions of the human body. It lies hidden, neither visible nor consciously noticeable in everyday life—yet it fulfills a central function. As the muscular "base plate" of the torso, it holds the organs in place, stabilizes the pelvis, controls the anal sphincter, and plays a major role in regulating abdominal pressure.

It is not a static structure, but a dynamic network of muscles that responds to every movement, every breath, and every inner tension. And for precisely this reason, it plays a key role in many complaints involving the lower abdomen and rectum—including hemorrhoids.

Supporting, bearing, counterbalancing

Normally, the pelvic floor works unnoticed. It contracts reflexively when we cough, sneeze, or lift heavy objects. It cushions pressure, ensures continence, and adapts to varying loads. But when it is overloaded, tense, or weakened, this balance can shift.

A chronic postural issue—for example, a tilted pelvis or prolonged sitting—can prevent the pelvic floor from fulfilling its supportive function. Instead of reacting flexibly, it may become too tight—or too slack. Both can disrupt pressure dynamics in the pelvic region and impair venous return from the rectum. The result: blood pools, veins dilate—and hemorrhoids can form or worsen.

Tension isn't always noticeable

What many don't realize is that excessive tension in the pelvic floor often isn't consciously felt. It doesn't always cause pain, but rather a subtle internal resistance, a feeling that "something's not right"—or it may show up in seemingly unrelated symptoms: constipation, a sensation of pressure, incomplete evacuation, or the feeling of "not fully being in control."

In my case, I only understood much later that my pelvic floor had been chronically active for years—likely compensating for an unstable pelvic alignment. This permanent tension wasn't consciously controllable. I couldn't "relax" because I wasn't even aware that I was tense. Only through targeted bodywork and focused attention on the deep muscle layers did I realize how overactive this area had become.

Breathing, posture, and relaxation

The pelvic floor works closely with the diaphragm, the deep abdominal muscles, and the back muscles. When breathing is shallow, the torso tense, or posture misaligned, the pelvic floor can no longer respond freely. It becomes a silent co-compensator for a constant imbalance—right in one of the body's most sensitive areas.

Conversely, this means that anyone who learns to breathe consciously, center their posture, and regulate the pelvic floor not forcefully but with subtlety, can achieve a great deal. Not through strength training—but through awareness, release, and the dissolution of unconscious tension.

A key often overlooked

Looking back, the pelvic floor was one of the most crucial factors in my healing process—though I only came to understand that later. It is neither the sole cause nor the only solution, but it is a central link: between posture and function, between internal and external perception, between tension and relief.

Anyone who regularly suffers from rectal issues should not treat the pelvic floor as a side note—but as a key junction. Not for training in the gym—but for understanding.

9.3 – Jaw Misalignments (CMD) and Their Impact on Body Posture

A connection hardly anyone suspects: when people talk about hemorrhoids, they think about digestion, diet, toilet habits—but almost no one thinks about the jaw. And yet it was precisely this part of the body that ultimately played a decisive role in my case. Many years after the initial symptoms, I was eventually diagnosed—through various detours—with a condition called craniomandibular dysfunction, or CMD for short.

CMD refers to a dysfunction or misalignment of the temporomandibular joint and its surrounding structures. It can trigger numerous symptoms: headaches, neck pain, tinnitus, teeth grinding, jaw clicking—and also postural changes that can extend all the way to the pelvic area.

What may initially sound far-fetched becomes quite logical upon closer inspection: the body is an interconnected system. If something is misaligned at the top—in the jaw—the rest of the body must compensate. And that has consequences.

The Chain of Effects: From Jaw to Pelvis

The temporomandibular joint is closely connected to the spine via muscular chains, fasciae, and neural pathways. Even a slight misalignment—caused by a high dental crown, nighttime clenching, or a tilted pelvis—can lead to chronic tension that reverberates throughout the body.

In my case, this manifested as a shifted pelvis, which went unnoticed for a long time. My body adapted, compensated, "made it work." But this constant compensation created pressure—on joints, muscles, and connective tissue. And that very pressure affects the rectal area too. When the pelvis is persistently tilted or twisted, it alters the pressure dynamics in the abdominal region—and with it the venous drainage from the hemorrhoidal area.

In my case, CMD was not just a side issue, but possibly a silent trigger—or at least a major aggravating factor of the condition.

The Great Invisibility of CMD

What makes things even more difficult is that CMD often goes undiagnosed. Many dentists pay little attention to jaw joint alignment during routine check-ups. And general practitioners or orthopedists rarely link pelvic or intestinal complaints with the jaw. Patients themselves often have no clue—because the symptoms appear unrelated.

It wasn't until I happened upon a holistically oriented dentist—who considered the body as a whole—that this connection even came up. And indeed: after the first targeted treatment of my jaw, combined with a custom-fitted bite splint, I noticed changes in my lower back. The chain began to loosen.

Posture Isn't Just Theory—It's Everyday Reality

Anyone who has ever walked around for a day with a slightly too short leg—perhaps due to an ill-fitting shoe—knows how quickly the body falls out of alignment. And how it can be felt everywhere. With CMD, this imbalance is permanent. The body compensates—day after day. And that constant counterbalancing creates tension—often in the deep pelvic area. Precisely where many assume it's only about diet or sitting habits.

CMD doesn't just affect the head—it impacts the entire body. And when you live long-term with a crooked foundation, it can eventually lead to problems—even in places you'd never expect.

Seeing the Whole Picture

For me, realizing that a jaw misalignment could contribute to hemorrhoids was a true aha moment. Not because it immediately solved all my problems—but because it finally established a logical connection. Between top and bottom. Between posture and symptom. Between cause and effect.

It was the moment I understood: if you truly want to change something, you must view the body as a whole—and not stop at the place where the pain just happens to show up.

9.4 – Personal Observations During My CMD Treatment

When I began treatment for CMD, my hemorrhoids were still far from any kind of improvement. Looking back, I would categorize them as grade three to four. The nodes were sometimes the size of cherries, clearly palpable—and they would prolapse regularly. It had become routine for me to push these bulges back in with one finger—sometimes even two. While I had become accustomed to this, it was by no means pleasant. It meant that the problem was constantly present—every day, with every movement, during every bathroom visit.

By that point, I had already undergone two surgeries, tried various conservative treatments—and yet I found myself right back at the beginning. It wasn't until I started splint therapy as part of my CMD treatment that I felt a sense of renewed hope for the first time.

The Splint Brings Relief—Slow but Noticeable

I started using a custom-made bite splint—initially at night, and later occasionally during the day. The goal was to reduce unconscious jaw tension and, in turn, regulate the body's entire tension chain. And while the process was subtle and slow, I began to notice a change.

After about six months, I had the impression that the hemorrhoids were becoming less noticeable. They were still present, but I didn't need to push them back in every day. The tissue seemed less irritated, the pressure decreased. It wasn't a dramatic breakthrough, but rather a gradual shift—in the right direction.

Additional Support: MUCOKEHL D3

Around the same time, I also began treating the affected area with a cream that had been recommended to me: MUCOKEHL D3 by Sanum Kehlbeck—an isopathic remedy that I'll describe in more detail later. I used the cream in addition to the CMD treatment—not as a standalone solution, but as part of a new, more holistic approach.

I applied it regularly, often in the evening—and felt that it contributed to a calming effect. The itching decreased, the tissue felt more regenerated. The remedy is also available in suppository form, but for me, the cream was sufficient. It felt like I had finally found a combination that didn't work against my body, but with it.

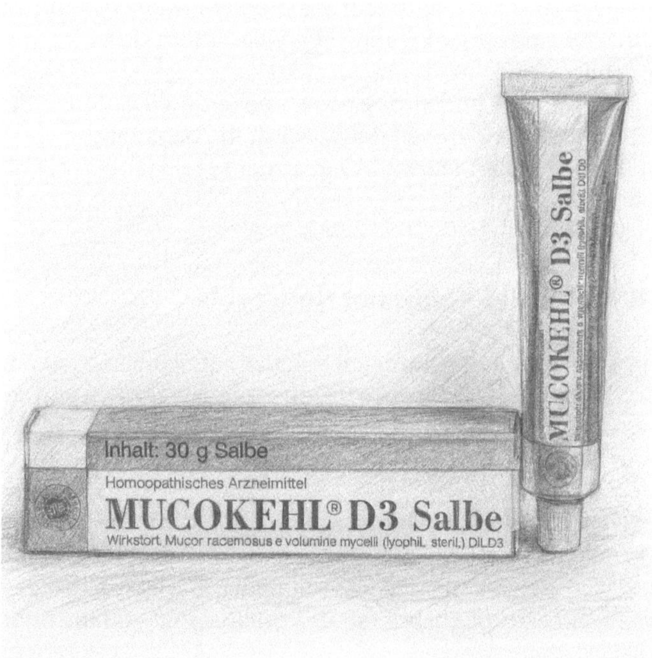

Gradual Reduction—Stable Progress

As my CMD treatment continued—especially during the first and second year—the positive effect became stronger. The hemorrhoids got smaller. At first, I was cautiously optimistic, but eventually it became clear: this was no longer just coincidence. The pressure diminished, and the tissue visibly receded. Today, several years after starting splint therapy, I would classify the condition as grade one to two—clearly improved, without any surgical interventions.

Today, I can live a mostly normal life—without daily discomfort, without constantly having to push anything back in, and without excessive caution during every toilet visit. Of course, I still monitor the situation carefully—but for the first time in many years, I feel like my body is no longer working against itself.

Insight: The Body Often Just Needs the Right Impulse

What this experience has shown me is that sometimes the body doesn't need drastic interventions—just the right kind of relief in the right place. In my case, it was the jaw—a hidden source of disruption that had been influencing my entire body's tension field. The combination of splint therapy, targeted body awareness, and supportive care achieved more than any surgery ever had.

Looking back, this development confirms what I now firmly believe: if you take the body seriously—if you listen, observe, and think systemically—you often discover entirely different paths to improvement. Paths that may take longer, but ultimately lead to more sustainable results.

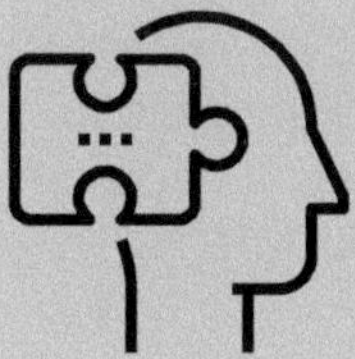

Did You Know…?

Many people affected by CMD (jaw joint dysfunction) simultaneously suffer from functional disorders in the pelvic region – through muscular chains, this can also affect the rectum.

Chapter 10 – Daily Life, Bowel Habits, and Lifestyle

After all the medical treatments and the exploration of posture, tension, and body alignment, I gradually realized that everyday life itself plays a major role—often underestimated, but consistently influential. Because what we do daily—how we sit, eat, walk, or use the toilet—shapes our body more than any short-term intervention ever could.

Section 10.1 focuses on prolonged sitting and lack of movement—a pattern that is widespread in our society. I describe how continuous sitting affects the pelvis, why it can hinder venous return, and what happens when the body doesn't get the balance it needs. Even small movement impulses can make a big difference here.

Section 10.2 addresses another often underestimated factor: chronic stress and its effect on the digestive system. The close connection between the nervous system and digestion—keyword: gut-brain axis—is particularly evident in functional disorders. I explain how I personally experienced this connection and why inner tension is often the invisible trigger for physical symptoms.

Section 10.3 explores a topic that may sound trivial at first but can have a significant impact: toilet posture—the difference between sitting and squatting. I share how I changed my posture during bowel movements and how much of a difference it made. From an anatomical perspective, squatting is the human body's natural position for elimination. Once you understand this, it becomes clear that even simple changes in daily habits can have powerful effects.

Chapter 10 shows: not everything requires therapy or medication. Sometimes it's enough to question your habits—and give your body back what originally did it good.

10.1 – Prolonged Sitting and Lack of Movement

Humans are not designed to spend the majority of their day sitting. Our bodies are built for movement—for walking, standing, squatting, carrying, bending. But the reality of modern life looks different: we sit in the car, at the office, during meals, while watching TV. Often for hours on end—in the same position. And that's exactly the problem.

Prolonged, static sitting doesn't just affect the back and muscles—it also directly impacts the pelvic region, venous return, and ultimately the sensitive structures around the rectum. Those who sit for long periods throw their entire pressure system out of balance. And this imbalance can contribute to the development or worsening of hemorrhoids.

The Pelvis in a Fixed Position – A Backup Begins

While sitting, the pelvis tilts slightly. Pressure is placed on the lower part of the pelvis, especially the coccyx and rectum. Most chair surfaces are not designed to distribute weight evenly—they compress instead. This impairs venous return from the pelvic area and causes blood to pool. The delicate vascular cushions in the anal canal are constantly stressed—a condition you hardly notice, but which silently does its damage.

If physical movement is also lacking, the natural impulses that activate the lymphatic system and venous pump are missing. Circulation slows, tension in the pelvic floor increases, and pressure in the lower abdomen becomes a permanent risk factor.

Lack of Movement Means Lack of Balance

Exercise is not just important for the heart and circulation—it's essential for the nourishment and relief of the entire trunk. Even light walking, standing, or stretching can help regulate pressure in the pelvis. When these stimuli are absent—such as in predominantly sedentary jobs—the body lacks balance. Bowel movements become sluggish, tissue becomes undernourished, and tension patterns in the pelvis continue to shift.

I didn't realize this in my own daily life for a long time. I spent hours working at a desk, driving, sitting on the couch in the evening. I would stand up now and then, but real movement was rare. Only in retrospect did I recognize how much these patterns had burdened my body over the years—without me ever noticing.

What Changes When You Start Moving

The good news: even small changes can have a big impact. Taking regular breaks, standing up in between, stretching, or walking for a few minutes brings the body back into motion. Even mindful sitting—on a wedge cushion, an exercise ball, or by varying positions—can noticeably reduce pressure on the pelvis.

Later, I began to intentionally incorporate movement into my day—not as a workout, but as a rhythm. A short walk, a few squats, a mobility exercise for the pelvis. The goal wasn't to become fit, but to become more open, more flexible. And that made a real difference.

Sitting Remains – But Not Inactively

Completely avoiding sitting is unrealistic for most people. But it's not about setting extreme rules. It's about not letting sitting become a permanent condition. About relieving the body regularly. About understanding movement not as a duty, but as a signal to the body: you may breathe again.

Today, I'm more mindful of these patterns. I notice more quickly when my body begins to "lock up." And I know now that many of my earlier symptoms weren't just about diet or genetics—but about inactivity. That may have been one of the simplest, yet most powerful realizations along this journey.

10.2 – Chronic Stress and Its Impact on the Gut

When the body stays in alarm mode: Stress isn't just a short-term phenomenon. When it becomes chronic, it turns into a state—a background tone in the body that affects everything: digestion, breathing, muscle tension, hormone balance, sleep quality, and pain perception. The gut, in particular, reacts sensitively to this constant internal state.

In stress mode—whether triggered by external pressure, internal tension, or unresolved conflicts—the body shifts its energy distribution: digestion is downregulated, blood flow is redirected, and muscle tension increases. While this response makes sense in acute danger, it becomes harmful when it turns into a long-term condition. The gut suffers.

Digestion requires relaxation

The activity of the intestines is closely linked to the parasympathetic nervous system—the part of our autonomic nervous system responsible for rest, regeneration, and digestion. In contrast, the sympathetic nervous system governs activity, performance, fight-or-flight responses, and constant tension.

As long as the body remains in sympathetic mode—as is often the case with chronic stress—digestion is inhibited. The gut becomes sluggish, irregular, and slow. At the same time, muscle tone in the abdominal and pelvic area increases. An internal pressure builds—often imperceptible and beyond conscious control—but it nonetheless affects bowel movements and the venous structures of the rectum.

Gut-brain axis: the second nervous system

What many people don't know: the gut has its own nervous system—the so-called enteric nervous system. It contains about as many nerve cells as the spinal cord and is often referred to as the "second brain." This system is in constant communication with the brain—via nerve pathways, neurotransmitters, and hormones.

This means: our thoughts, worries, fears, and inner tensions have a direct effect on the gut. Conversely, the condition of the gut influences our mood, irritability, and perception of stress. It's a reciprocal relationship that has long been underestimated in conventional medicine—but is now increasingly researched.

My own experience with stress and digestion

Looking back, I can say clearly: during the most stressful periods of my life—such as work-related pressure, family crises, or personal uncertainty—my digestive system was also at its most vulnerable. I felt tense, restless, and driven. And during exactly these times, my hemorrhoids were at their worst.

It was a recurring pattern. My digestion slowed, bowel movements became more strained, and pushing things back in became more difficult. Only with more rest, conscious relief, and inner stability did I feel physical relaxation again. Eventually, the connection became impossible to ignore.

Slowing down as therapy

Of course, you can't simply "switch off" stress. But you can learn to recognize it—and consciously counteract it. Whether through breathing exercises, walks, open conversations, more sleep, reduced media consumption, or regular breaks—anything that calms the nervous system also benefits the gut, and by extension, the entire pelvic area.

For me, this insight was another key: hemorrhoids are not just a tissue issue—they're also a matter of inner posture. Anyone who goes through life constantly tense will sooner or later receive physical warning signs. The gut is one of the first to speak.

The real question is: are we listening?

10.3 – Toilet Culture: The Difference Between Sitting and Squatting

The way we use the toilet is something most people take for granted—shaped by cultural standards, design habits, and architectural norms. But what is considered "normal" today in Western countries—namely, bowel movements while sitting on a toilet seat—is far from ideal from an anatomical perspective.

From a medical standpoint, the human body is originally designed for the squatting position. In a deep squat, the angle of the intestines straightens, the pelvic floor relaxes, and the pressure flow from the colon to the anus becomes more natural. Elimination becomes easier, more complete, and requires less straining. This last point is particularly important—especially for people with hemorrhoids.

The anorectal angle – a small detail with a big impact

When sitting, a so-called anorectal angle forms between the rectum and the anal canal. This kink helps maintain continence while at rest—which is beneficial—but it also impedes flow during defecation. To overcome this angle, many people feel the need to strain. And that straining increases pressure on the sensitive hemorrhoidal cushions.

In a squatting position, however, this angle almost fully straightens. Natural gravity supports the process, pressure on the rectum is more evenly distributed, and the pelvic floor can relax more effectively. It's a combination of posture, breathing, and muscular tension that noticeably relieves the body—during a process we go through several times a day.

My own transition – a small change with big results

About three years ago, I started to consciously change my toilet posture. Since then, I've used a footstool that raises my feet during bowel movements—creating a near-squat position. It has now become completely natural for me not to "do my business" in the conventional seated way.

What felt unfamiliar at first quickly became routine—and in retrospect, it made a noticeable contribution to easing my symptoms. Alongside other measures—such as CMD treatment, supportive ointments, improved bowel habits, and more mindful posture—this change was another small but crucial step in giving my body what it originally needs.

Culture vs. body logic

Western toilet culture is a product of modernity—comfortable, hygienic, standardized. But what was invented for the sake of convenience doesn't necessarily meet the body's functional needs. In many other cultures, squatting is still the common defecation position—and for good reason.

Of course, no one needs to completely remodel their bathroom. Often, a simple footstool, a small platform—or just the awareness of how much a slight shift in position can aid elimination—is enough. What matters isn't perfection, but direction.

Conclusion: Relief begins with the angle

Today I'm convinced: switching to a squatting position was one of the most practical and effective steps toward a life with fewer symptoms. It cost nothing, required no medication—just the willingness to question ingrained habits.

Anyone suffering from hemorrhoids or who often feels "not quite emptied" should not underestimate this aspect. The body will cooperate—if we allow it to function in the natural way it was designed to.

Chapter 11 – Fascia, Nerves, and Muscular Tension

Anyone who deals with chronic issues like hemorrhoids over a longer period will eventually come across terms like fascia, tension patterns, or neural signaling pathways. While these may initially sound esoteric or overly complex, they turn out—on closer inspection—to be a key to understanding how the body works. Because our body is not a loose collection of parts, but a connected system of tension and signals, in which everything is linked to everything else.

In the first section, **Chapter 11.1**, we look at the fascial structures: the connective tissue-like layers and sheaths that surround and interconnect our muscles, organs, and nerves. Often overlooked, these structures can play a far greater role in chronic complaints than one might think—especially when they become stuck together or remain under constant tension.

In **Chapter 11.2**, we explore how tension is transmitted through the body—for example, from the jaw to the back, or from the back to the pelvis. Especially in my own case, where CMD (jaw joint dysfunction) played a central role, this connection was crucial: many symptoms in the anal region cannot be viewed in isolation but are often the result of misaligned posture and cascading tension chains throughout the body.

The next section, **Chapter 11.3**, takes a practical turn: What can I personally do to release tension? I introduce simple, everyday exercises that I've had good experiences with—not esoteric rituals, but small acts of mindfulness that can be easily integrated into daily life.

And finally, in **Chapter 11.4**, I describe the tangible improvements I experienced over time. The key insight: sometimes it's not the next surgery that brings a breakthrough—but rather the patient, systematic work on the root causes within your own body.

This chapter is therefore an invitation: to move away from purely symptom-focused thinking—and toward a deeper understanding of the body's internal interconnections, which often only become visible upon closer examination.

11.1 – Why Fascial Structures Matter

For many, the word fascia may initially sound like a trendy buzzword from the fitness world. But in reality, fasciae are a central element of our body. Fasciae are connective tissue sheaths and layers that stretch like a fine web throughout the entire body. They envelop muscles, organs, joints, and blood vessels—ensuring that everything is connected while still remaining mobile.

For a long time, they were regarded in medicine merely as packaging—largely ignored and often simply cut through during surgery. Only in recent years has research begun to understand just how active and important this tissue truly is. Because fasciae not only stabilize, but can also store tension, transmit it, and even sense pain.

From Local Symptoms to Global Tension

In my own case, it took me a long time to realize just how significantly fascial tension can affect the entire body. For years, I had issues in the pelvic area—and naturally, I first assumed local causes: mucous membranes, blood vessels, diet, sitting habits. But at some point, I began asking myself: why does the pressure keep returning? Why does it sometimes "pull" into my lower back, even though nothing seems to have changed in the rectum?

The answer lay—quite literally—in between: in the connective tissue that links everything. When fascial pathways are under tension, when the tissue becomes hardened, stuck, or permanently contracted, a tension pattern emerges that stretches across entire regions of the body. Depending on the course of these lines, this can also place pressure on the pelvic floor, the sacrum, and the surrounding structures.

Fasciae Are Not Rigid Tissue – They Are a Sensory Organ

What many people don't know is that fasciae are highly sensory-active. They contain more receptors than many other types of tissue. This means they perceive pressure, stretch, temperature changes—and transmit this information to the nervous system.

When under constant strain, poor posture, or emotional stress, the tissue may begin to "close off." It becomes less elastic, less permeable—and starts to pull at the body like a suit that's too tight.

In my case, this was probably a key factor: chronically overloaded connective tissue in the lower back and pelvic region that was constantly under tension, indirectly disrupting venous outflow. Not a blood congestion in the classic sense, but a mechanical imbalance—not originating in an organ, but in the tissue framework that holds everything together.

The Body Functions as a Whole – Not in Parts

Realizing that fasciae play an active role fundamentally changed my understanding of physical complaints. Suddenly, many things made more sense: why certain movements brought relief, why targeted stretching and "letting go" had more effect than medication, and why I always felt my symptoms worsened whenever my entire body was tense—not just locally, but systemically.

Fasciae connect—both literally and figuratively. They form bridges between muscles and joints, but also between various symptoms. They store posture, tension, and often even old injuries or emotional patterns. That's why it's worth paying attention to them—especially when dealing with symptoms that can't be clearly localized or explained.

A New Perspective on Old Complaints

Looking back, I'm convinced that I would never have truly understood the physical component of my issues without including fascial structures. For years, I had searched for a single cause—but there wasn't just one trigger. It was a network of tension that had gradually built up.

Today, I no longer see fasciae as a buzzword, but as the body's interconnected communication system. And anyone who begins thinking in terms of these connections—instead of just symptoms—often uncovers patterns that were previously hidden.

11.2 – Tension Transmission in the Body: Jaw, Back, Pelvis

When we talk about "posture," most people think of the back, shoulders, or perhaps the neck. What's often forgotten, however, is that patterns of tension act across long distances—not randomly, but along clearly defined pathways. Muscles, fasciae, and the nervous system don't work in isolation; they function in coordinated chains. When you create tension at the top, a reaction often occurs below—and vice versa.

This helps explain why symptoms in the anal or rectal area—such as hemorrhoids—are sometimes connected to entirely different regions of the body than one might expect. The jaw, the spine, and the pelvis, in particular, are closely—and often underestimatedly—interconnected.

The Jaw as a Source of Tension

In my case, it was the jaw that eventually set many things in motion—literally and figuratively. Due to a condition known as craniomandibular dysfunction (CMD), which I had unknowingly carried for many years, my bite was slightly misaligned. This minimal imbalance had tangible effects: it caused persistent tension in the jaw muscles, which radiated through the neck, shoulders, and back—all the way to the pelvis.

The fascial network and muscle chains transmit this tension—especially along what's known as the superficial back line, which extends from the top of the head to the soles of the feet. So, if there's "too much pressure" in the jaw, it can travel down the spine, reaching the sacrum and pelvic floor. There, it disrupts the fine balance between supportive and relaxing musculature, which can ultimately affect the venous structures of the rectum.

The Back as a Tension Conduit

The spine is not just a support structure—it's a kind of central tension and reaction hub for the body. Any imbalance, muscular asymmetry, or prolonged one-sided posture creates a kind of "tension storage" along the spine. The lower back—especially the lumbar spine and sacrum—is particularly affected when the body falls out of alignment.

For a long time, I didn't notice this in daily life. I had no classic back pain—but I felt a constant downward pull, a kind of pressure in the pelvic area that I couldn't quite place. Today, I understand: this wasn't "just" a symptom, but a result of tension that had built up and been stored over years—and eventually manifested in the body's most sensitive zone.

The Pelvis as a Central Junction

The pelvis is the link between the upper body and the legs—physically and functionally. Many tension fields converge here: the upright posture of the spine, the propulsion from walking, the work of the pelvic floor, the mobility of the hips. When one of these areas is chronically blocked—due to uneven posture, a tight back, or a tilted pelvis—tension isn't "resolved." It's transmitted or "deposited" elsewhere.

In my case, many issues manifested in the pelvic region: excessive tension, unconscious holding, restricted mobility. All of this made it harder for pressure to be released—leading to effects on the hemorrhoidal area. Only when I began to view the body system as a whole did I realize how crucial this connection truly is.

Thinking in Lines, Not Zones

One of the most important insights for me was this: the body doesn't function in zones—it works in lines. Pain or pressure often appears where it "arrives," not where it originates. The jaw tightens—the back compensates—the pelvis takes over—and ultimately, the most sensitive part suffers: the rectum.

This tension transmission isn't always perceptible—but it's real. And it explains why local treatments sometimes fail to produce lasting relief—because the root cause doesn't lie at the site of the symptom.

Releasing Tension—The Right Way

Today, I pay much closer attention to my overall tension state. I no longer just ask: Where does it hurt?, but also: Where am I holding on? Where do I carry tension that doesn't even belong to me? Where does what I feel really begin?

This new body awareness has changed a lot for me. Not through dramatic exercises or complicated therapies—but through the simple, consistent understanding of how things are connected.

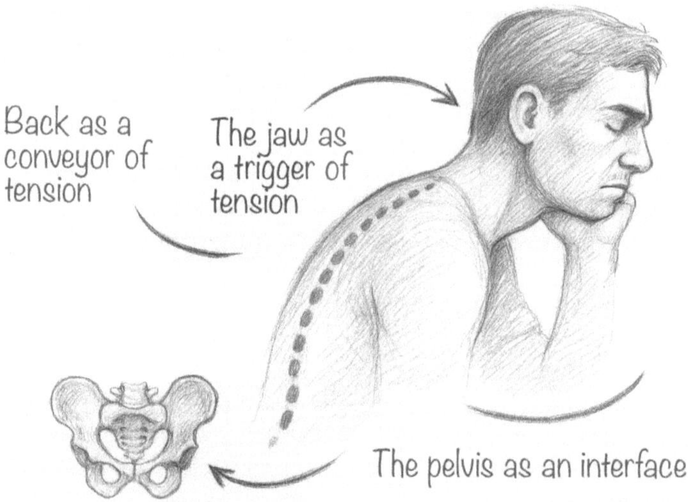

11.3 – Exercises for Conscious Relaxation

Many chronic complaints don't arise from isolated postural issues or injuries, but rather from ongoing states of tension that we no longer even notice in daily life. The body becomes accustomed to a certain baseline tension—and often only realizes something is out of balance through the appearance of pain. This is where targeted relaxation exercises come in: they not only help us regain physical balance, but also improve our body awareness.

Below, I'd like to share a few simple but effective exercises that were especially helpful to me during my own healing journey. They're not a "cure," but they can be an important part of a sustainable recovery.

1. Consciously Relax the Jaw

This exercise is simple but powerful:

- Sit calmly and close your eyes.
- Notice how your teeth are meeting. Do you feel pressure?
- Let your lower jaw slowly drop. Keep your lips gently closed.
- Imagine your jaw becoming soft, like wax melting in the sun.
- Breathe deeply in and out. With each exhale, let a little more tension go.

This exercise can be done several times a day—especially during stressful moments or while working at a desk.

2. Micro-Movements in the Pelvis

The pelvis is often a "blind spot" in body awareness. Small movements can help reconnect to that area:

- Sit on a chair with a firm seat.
- Gently tilt your pelvis forward and backward.
- Feel how your sit bones shift.
- Imagine your pelvis as a boat rocking on gentle waves.

Do these movements slowly and mindfully for 1–2 minutes.

3. Fascia Release with a Tennis Ball

Simple tools can help release deep-seated tension:

Lie on the floor and place a tennis ball under one side of your gluteal muscles.

- Slowly shift your weight onto the ball until you feel a gentle pressure.
- Move in small circles or stay still on a tight spot.
- Breathe into the tension consciously.
- After 1–2 minutes, switch sides.

This technique also works well for the lower back or hamstrings.

4. Nerve Stretch (Butler Method)

Many symptoms are caused by irritated or tense nerve pathways. A gentle stretch can help:

- Lie on your back, one leg extended, the other bent.
- Raise the bent leg toward the ceiling, hold it under the knee, and gently pull it toward your torso.
- Carefully flex your foot, as if trying to touch the ceiling with your heel.
- Hold the stretch for 10–15 seconds, then release.

This exercise is particularly helpful for sciatic issues or pelvic floor tension.

5. Breathing Exercise for Full-Body Relaxation

Breathing is the key to inner calm and physical release:

- Lie on your back or sit comfortably.
- Inhale slowly while counting to four.
- Hold your breath for two seconds.
- Exhale slowly while counting to six.
- Pause again briefly.

Repeat this five to ten times. You'll notice: with each repetition, your overall body tension decreases.

Conclusion on Relaxation Exercises

Relaxation isn't a luxury—it's an active strategy for self-regulation. Especially with chronic conditions like hemorrhoids, which are often linked to unclear body patterns, targeted exercises can help restore a new sense of balance. What matters is not how long or intensely you practice, but how mindfully and regularly.

The body remembers everything. And it changes—if we give it the chance.

Chapter 12 – The Role of Nutrition and Gut Health

When it comes to the development, treatment, and prevention of hemorrhoids, the role of nutrition is often mentioned—but rarely fully understood. In many conversations, articles, and self-help guides, we're advised to "eat more fiber" or "drink plenty of fluids." But what does that actually mean? And how exactly does nutrition affect our digestion, our bowel movements, and ultimately our risk of developing hemorrhoids?

This chapter explores that very connection. It's a topic that has accompanied me for many years—sometimes just in the background, sometimes with full awareness. Through my own experiences, I've learned that nutrition isn't a cure-all, but it's a key component that can meaningfully complement many other measures. What fascinated me most was how small changes in everyday habits often had a greater effect than expensive medications or therapies.

Chapter 12.1 focuses on fiber—those often underrated components of our diet that keep the digestive system running. I'll explain where to find them, what they do, and how they can be used in targeted ways—for example, with psyllium husks or specific foods.

Chapter 12.2 looks at hydration and stool consistency. This is another often underestimated factor: people who don't drink enough water tend to have hard stools—and those put unnecessary strain on the hemorrhoidal vessels. The body is a system, and every part of it affects the others.

In **Chapter 12.3**, I turn to the microbiome—our gut flora—as well as probiotics and the general composition of the intestinal environment. Although my personal experience with this area has been mixed, I still believe it's important not to ignore it—since for many others, it can play a much more significant role.

Finally, **Chapter 12.4** offers a personal look at what I've implemented in my own everyday life—simple habits with noticeable impact. My daily muesli ritual, a few basic guidelines, and the realization that consistency is often more important than perfection. This chapter doesn't end with dogmas, but with encouraging insights: nutrition is no mystery—it's something we can influence every single day.

12.1 – Fiber and Its Effect on Digestion

What exactly is fiber? Fiber refers to indigestible components of plant-based foods. That means our body can't break them down into nutrients or absorb them—but that's precisely what makes them so valuable. In the digestive system, they perform a number of supportive functions without being "used up" in the process.

There are two main types of fiber: soluble and insoluble. Soluble fiber absorbs water and swells—this increases stool volume and softens its consistency. Insoluble fiber, on the other hand, stimulates bowel movement (peristalsis) by mechanically irritating the intestinal lining and promoting forward motion of the food mass.

Why is fiber so important for hemorrhoids?

A common trigger for hemorrhoid issues is hard, dry stool. This leads to excessive straining during bowel movements—and that pressure puts significant stress on the delicate vascular cushions in the anal area. Over time, if these structures are constantly overburdened, hemorrhoids may develop or worsen.

Fiber helps make stool softer and easier to pass. This significantly reduces the need to strain during bowel movements—thereby relieving pressure on the hemorrhoidal tissue. For me personally, increasing my fiber intake was one of the first steps that made a noticeable difference.

Where can you find fiber?

Fiber is present in many natural foods, such as:

- **Whole grain products** (e.g. oats, whole grain bread, brown rice)
- **Legumes** (e.g. lentils, beans, chickpeas)
- **Vegetables** (e.g. carrots, broccoli, celery, cabbage)
- **Fruits** (e.g. apples, berries, pears—especially with the peel)
- **Nuts and seeds** (e.g. flaxseeds, chia seeds, sunflower seeds)

One particularly practical option is psyllium husks—a pure, natural product with an extremely high fiber content. They can absorb up to 40 times their own weight in water and are excellent for gently regulating digestion.

Psyllium husks as a targeted supplement

I've personally had very good experiences with psyllium husk powder. The best way to take it is about half an hour before a meal: stir one teaspoon into a large glass of water and drink it immediately. Very important: drink plenty of additional water afterward! Without enough fluids, the husks can clump in the gut and have the opposite of the intended effect. For many people, psyllium husks are a simple and inexpensive way to support their digestion—especially when combined with a more conscious diet.

Conclusion on fiber

Fiber isn't a miracle cure—but it is a fundamental building block of healthy digestion. Anyone who wants to reduce their hemorrhoid symptoms over the long term will find it hard to avoid. And the best part: it's easy to incorporate into everyday life—without major lifestyle changes or sacrifices.

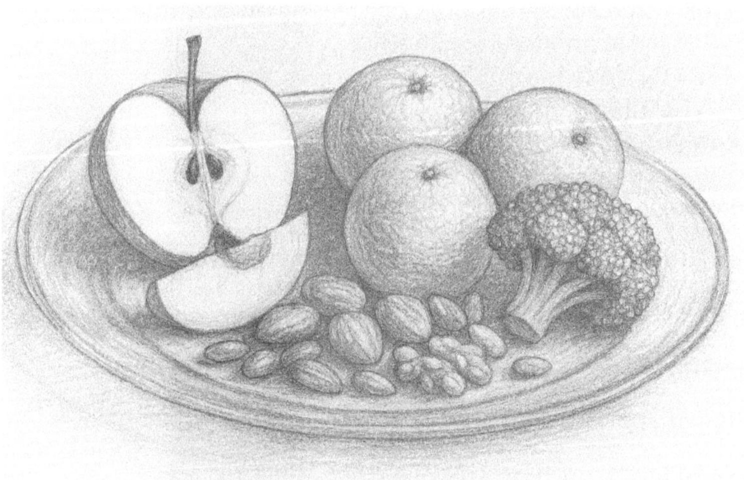

12.2 – Water Balance and Stool Consistency

Even though it may sound trivial, water balance plays a central role in our digestion—and thus also in the development or relief of hemorrhoids. The human body consists largely of water, and the intestines rely on an adequate supply of fluids to keep the food mass moving smoothly. If this fluid is lacking, the stool becomes harder and drier—making it more difficult to pass. This often leads to unnecessary straining, which increases pressure on the sensitive tissue in the rectal area and promotes or worsens hemorrhoids.

Hard facts about hard stool

Many sufferers report that they "go to the bathroom every day" and therefore assume that everything is fine. But frequency alone tells us very little. The consistency of the stool is far more important. Stool that is too hard or lumpy—often a result of dehydration—increases friction and mechanical resistance during bowel movements. This puts particular strain on the rectum.

A common pattern is sluggish bowel movements in the morning or after prolonged sitting—often showing up as small, firm pellets or very thick stool. Many interpret this as "normal" because they've experienced it for years. But in reality, it's a sign of a chronically suboptimal fluid balance—or an imbalanced diet.

How much water is enough?

The often-quoted recommendation to drink two to three liters of water per day isn't wrong—but it doesn't take individual differences into account. People who sweat a lot, are physically active, or consume a high-fiber diet may need more. What matters is not just the total amount, but whether the body receives fluids regularly throughout the day. In other words, more isn't always better—what's more important is consistent hydration.

A good indicator is the color of your urine: If it's light and clear, your body is likely well hydrated. Dark or strongly scented urine, on the other hand, can be a sign of dehydration—which also affects the digestive system.

Drinking alone isn't enough

It also matters what you drink. Coffee, black tea, or alcohol tend to have a dehydrating effect and shouldn't be counted toward your fluid intake. Ideal choices include still water, herbal teas, or diluted fruit juice spritzers. Water-rich foods like cucumbers, melons, or zucchini can also contribute to hydration.

Equally important: Fiber needs water to work properly. So if you're taking something like psyllium husks without enough fluids, you may end up causing the exact opposite of what you intended—constipation. That's why every fiber-rich meal should always be accompanied by adequate fluid intake.

Conclusion: Fluids as daily medicine

A stable water balance is not a miracle cure—but it is a basic prerequisite for healthy, smooth bowel movements. Anyone suffering from hemorrhoids, or looking to prevent them, should ensure a steady and conscious intake of fluids. It's one of the simplest and most effective measures—and at the same time, one of the most commonly overlooked in everyday life.

12.3 – Microbiome, Probiotics, and the Gut Environment

The human gut is home to billions of microorganisms—bacteria, fungi, and other tiny life forms that together make up what's known as the microbiome. This microbiome is not a static construct, but rather a highly dynamic system that responds daily to diet, stress, medication, and other environmental influences. A healthy gut flora contributes to digestion, immune defense, and even mood regulation. Conversely, a disrupted microbiome can encourage a range of issues—from bloating to chronic inflammation or skin problems.

Probiotics – Cure-all or Commercial Hype?

In the public eye, probiotics—supplements containing live "beneficial" gut bacteria—are often regarded as a kind of miracle cure. In theory, they're meant to support or rebalance the microbiome, especially after antibiotic treatments or during digestive troubles. There are indeed studies that support certain mechanisms of action. In practice, however, the effects are highly individual.

I've tried various probiotic regimens in the past myself. Some of them were quite expensive—and honestly, I noticed little to no effect. No noticeable improvement, except that I had 30 euros less in my wallet. That doesn't mean these products are generally ineffective—but it does show that one shouldn't expect miracles. What works for one person may do nothing for another. The microbiome is complex—and its response is not always predictable.

Stool Testing for Orientation

At one point, I did a stool test to gain more clarity. The result was surprisingly unspectacular: no major irregularities; according to the lab, the microbial environment was "relatively balanced." So I had no obvious reason to take further action—and set the topic aside again for a while.

Diet Remains the Key Factor

Regardless of specific supplements, one thing still holds true: diet is key. Those who eat a fiber-rich diet, largely avoid sugar and heavily processed foods, and regularly consume fresh vegetables and fermented foods are already doing their gut environment a big favor. Adequate hydration, regular physical activity, and stress reduction also play an important role.

Fermented products such as sauerkraut, kefir, plain yogurt, or kombucha contain natural microorganisms that can benefit the gut—without the need for capsules or powders. Personally, I didn't experience a dramatic effect from these either, but for many people, they're simply part of a healthy lifestyle.

Conclusion: No Miracle, but Worth Exploring

The topic of the microbiome is still the subject of intense research. Much remains unclear, and some claims are likely overstated. But one thing is certain: a healthy gut relies on a diverse bacterial population. Those who suffer from ongoing digestive issues or hemorrhoids may want to look into this area—ideally with professional guidance and without falling for marketing promises. For me, it wasn't a gamechanger—but I now see it as one more small piece in the bigger puzzle.

12.4 – Practical Nutrition Tips from Personal Experience

The Power of Small Rituals:

Among all the complex advice about nutrition, fiber, the microbiome, and gut health, it's often the simple, repeatable routines that make the biggest difference. In my case, it was especially a fixed breakfast ritual that proved itself over the years—not spectacular, but effective.

My Daily Breakfast: Muesli with Everything That Does Me Good

For quite some time now, I've started every day the same way: with a homemade muesli mixed with plain yogurt. I add a combination of:

- fresh fruit (depending on the season—e.g., apple, banana, berries),
- flax seeds,
- chia seeds,
- sunflower seeds, and
- walnuts.

This mix provides not only plenty of fiber but also healthy fats, protein, and valuable phytonutrients. At the same time, it's easy to digest and gives me the feeling of doing something good for my body right from the start of the day.

What's nice about it: This breakfast is neither complicated nor expensive. It can be varied as needed and takes only a few minutes to prepare. For me, it's a simple but steady component that does me good—without major experimentation.

Psyllium Husk as Additional Support

If you suffer from hard or irregular bowel movements, you can supplement your diet with psyllium husk powder. These small fibers have an extremely high swelling capacity and can make stool softer and bulkier—provided you drink enough water with them.

Application is simple: Stir one teaspoon of psyllium husks into a glass of water, drink it about half an hour before a meal, and follow up with another glass of water. It's crucial to drink plenty—otherwise, the effect can backfire. For me, psyllium was especially helpful during sluggish digestion phases—such as after surgery or during extended periods of stress.

Sometimes Less Is More

Apart from this breakfast and the occasional use of psyllium husks, I haven't followed any complex diets. I largely avoid heavily processed foods, make sure I drink enough water, and generally skip things like spicy seasonings or hard-to-digest fats—simply because I've found that they don't agree with me.

This rather intuitive approach has proven more sustainable for me than rigid meal plans. It wasn't about doing everything perfectly—but about doing the right things consistently.

Conclusion: Nutrition as a Foundation—Not a Substitute

A mindful diet can have a significant impact—especially with chronic conditions like hemorrhoids. But it does not replace identifying root causes. For me, the muesli became an important building block, but just one of many. Combined with movement, posture, relaxation, and targeted therapy, it formed a complete picture—and ultimately led to noticeable improvement.

1 2 3 4 5 6 7 8 9 10 11 12 13 14 15 16 A

Part 4: Paths to Relief – What Helps in the Long Run

Chapter 13 – Ointments, Baths, and Proven Remedies

When there's burning, itching, or pain in the anal area, many sufferers instinctively reach for what's most easily available: ointments, creams, suppositories, or sitz baths. Pharmacy and drugstore shelves are full of such products – and at first glance, the variety can be reassuring. After all, there must be something you can "just try out" that will help. But the truth is often more sobering: many of these remedies provide short-term symptom relief but fail to address the root cause. And quite often, they mark the beginning of a long journey through a maze of promises, disappointments, and a lingering feeling of not being taken seriously.

This chapter offers an honest overview: What can over-the-counter products actually do – and what can't they? Which remedies have personally worked for me, and which ones felt like little more than a damp squib? I openly share my experiences with ointments like MUCOKEHL D3, classic zinc creams, and even an unusual Chinese ointment with a strong musk scent – which, surprisingly, turned out to be quite effective. This is not about advertising, but about sharing real-world experience. Because when you're suffering long-term, you don't want theory – you want practical advice that can truly make a difference.

Another focus of this chapter is sitz baths – especially after surgical procedures, they can offer real relief. I personally used them regularly only in the immediate post-op period, and at that time, I found them genuinely helpful. After that, to be honest, I quickly stopped using them. Still, I want to include them here, as they are a standard part of many treatment approaches and – when used correctly – absolutely have their place.

Finally, we'll look at a topic few like to discuss: relapses. They can be frustrating, but for many, they're simply part of the healing journey. A calm, clear-minded approach is essential here – along with the realization that you don't have to function perfectly every single day. If you see a relapse not as a failure, but as your body's signal, you stay in control – and empowered to act.

A short section also touches on a question many eventually ask: Surgery – yes or no? I'm not here to offer a recommendation, but a nudge for reflection. Because surgery is a serious decision. It shouldn't be postponed out of fear – but also not rushed into out of impatience.

13.1 What Over-the-Counter Products Can Do

For most people experiencing hemorrhoids for the first time, the natural response is to reach for what's readily available: over-the-counter ointments, suppositories, sitz baths, or herbal remedies from the pharmacy. The selection is vast, and the promises on the packaging sound convincing – but what can these products actually achieve?

Relief, Not a Cure

Over-the-counter remedies are primarily aimed at relieving acute symptoms: itching, burning, oozing, or a mild pressure sensation. The active ingredients are often anti-inflammatory, astringent (tissue-tightening), or mildly numbing. Common substances include witch hazel, lidocaine, zinc oxide, or aloe vera. Herbal combinations featuring horse chestnut or chamomile are also frequently used.

Effectiveness: Limited and Often Temporary

In the short term, these products can indeed offer some relief. Burning may subside, itching can decrease, and minor irritation may calm down. However, what they usually don't offer is a lasting solution to the problem. Ointments and creams work on the surface – they don't address the root cause. Those hoping for a miracle drug from the drugstore that will permanently eliminate their symptoms are often disappointed.

What's more, the effects of many of these remedies are rather subtle. It may take several days to notice any improvement – if at all. Some preparations show no noticeable effect, and many sufferers find themselves switching from one product to another in frustration, hoping to finally "find something that works." This can quickly lead to feelings of dependence or uncertainty, especially in the early stages.

Unconventional Options from the Kitchen Cabinet

In some cases, people report unusual alternatives. Pure olive oil, for example, is occasionally mentioned as a gentle, non-irritating treatment. It moisturizes the skin, can produce a soothing sensation when applied, and contains natural antioxidants.

Of course, it's not a medical cure – but sometimes even a simple, natural substance is enough to bring temporary relief.

Overall, over-the-counter products can be a helpful first aid – especially if you're dealing with acute discomfort or are unsure how serious the issue really is. However, they're rarely sufficient as a long-term solution. If you want to stay symptom-free in the long run, you need to broaden your perspective – toward diet, movement, body awareness, and overall lifestyle.

Because hemorrhoids are rarely just a skin problem – they are often a sign of a deeper imbalance in the entire system.

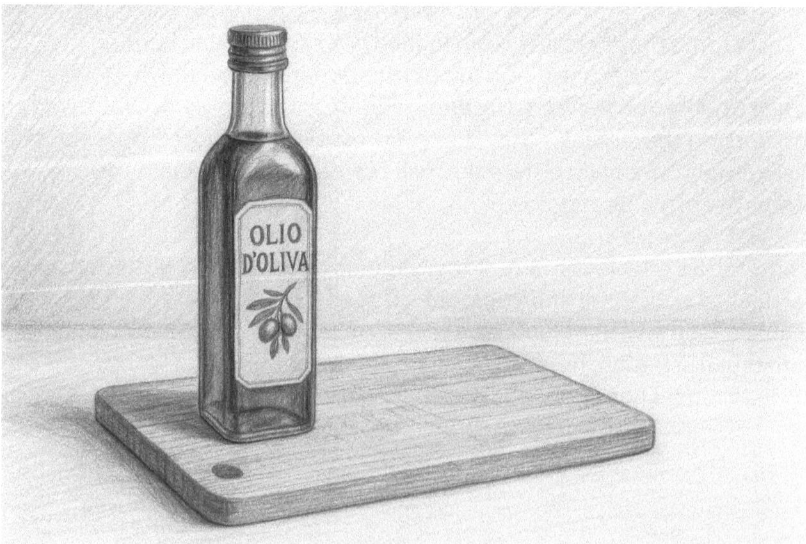

13.2 Personally Tested Remedies and Their Effects

MUCOKEHL D3: The One Remedy That Truly Helped

After trying many different products, there was ultimately only one that brought lasting improvement to my hemorrhoids: MUCOKEHL D3 ointment by Sanum Kehlbeck. It belongs to a form of treatment known as isopathic therapy – a method similar to homeopathy, but more differentiated and targeted. The active ingredient, Mucokehl, is derived from components of a specific mold (Mucor racemosus) and is believed to have a strong regulatory effect on connective tissue and vascular walls.

- A biological remedy with an isopathic component that works holistically
- Regulates mucous membranes and influences the internal environment (something conventional medicine doesn't even consider)
- Available in suppository form for deeper effects → often ideal for internal hemorrhoids

Whether or not you believe in these kinds of therapies – in my case, the result was clearly positive. While many other remedies only provided temporary relief, MUCOKEHL was the first one that made me feel like the tissue was truly regenerating and something was changing on a deeper level.

It's easy to use: apply it regularly, especially internally, ideally after a bowel movement and proper cleaning. I used it over several months – not in a state of panic, but consistently and calmly. And that, it seems, made all the difference.

Pasta Zinci Molli: Classic Zinc Ointment for Irritation Relief

Also helpful – though more in the acute stage – was Pasta Zinci Molli, a classic zinc ointment that can be custom-compounded at a pharmacy. It has mild anti-inflammatory properties, soothes irritated skin, and forms a light protective barrier. Especially for weeping or slightly inflamed areas, this can be very pleasant.

However, its effect is purely superficial and usually lasts only as long as the ointment remains on the skin. It wasn't a solution for long-term healing in my case – but as a temporary support, it's definitely recommendable.

One downside of zinc ointments: they tend to leave white stains on clothing, which is why I used this remedy rather sparingly.

Ma Ying Long: The Chinese Method with Deep Effect

A more exotic but truly noteworthy remedy is Ma Ying Long Musk Hemorrhoid Cream – a traditional Chinese product available via eBay or Amazon. Its scent is intense, almost pungent – classic musk, blended with essential oils and herbal extracts. The cream produces a pleasantly cooling effect and initially calms the area.

- Used for decades in Asia
- Anti-inflammatory, decongestant, cooling
- Strong local effect thanks to musk and herbal extracts
- Acts locally, not systemically – directly at the problem site
- Ideal for early to moderate stages

What makes this cream truly unique is its ability to deliberately irritate the tissue, which, after a few days, can lead to regression or even the detachment of small hemorrhoidal parts. In a way, it resembles a minimally invasive treatment like sclerotherapy or rubber band ligation – but purely external. In my own case, a mild burning sensation developed after several days – and eventually, a small piece of tissue actually detached.

The application follows a cyclical pattern: apply once or twice daily until a piece of tissue detaches. After that, it is advisable to take a break for a few days to allow the area to recover before beginning the next round.

Prospective use as a staged treatment concept

I could imagine using this ointment as the first step in a two-stage treatment system for severe hemorrhoids – followed by a transition to MUCOKEHL D3. The idea would be to treat the external hemorrhoids with Ma Ying Long over the course of several weeks, and then, once visible regression has occurred, continue working "inward" over the following months using MUCOKEHL D3.

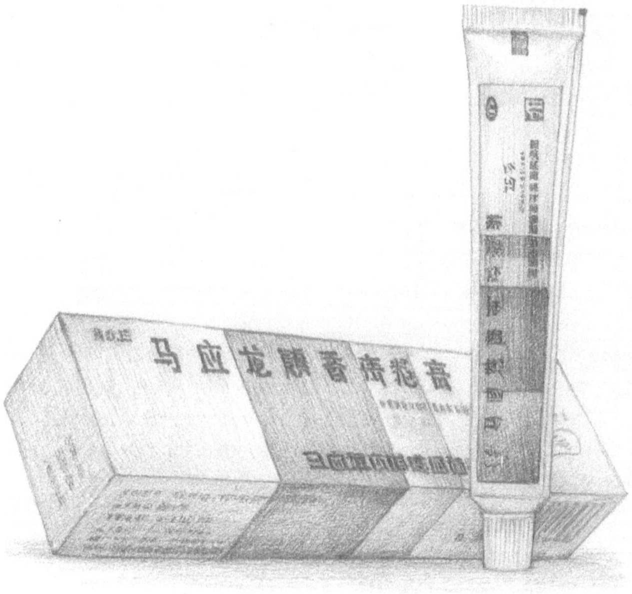

Conclusion: Try – But Not Blindly

These three remedies accompanied me over many years – some for longer, some only briefly. One thing is clear: not every product works the same for everyone. But if you observe yourself attentively and avoid overuse, you can often sense what your body responds to – and what it doesn't.

For me personally, the best approach was a combination of one truly deep-acting remedy (MUCOKEHL) and occasional supportive care (zinc ointment or olive oil).

Exotic treatments like the Ma Ying Long cream can be an interesting addition – but they should be used mindfully and not just out of curiosity or desperation.

In the end, the most important insight remains: Patience, self-observation, and consistency beat any miracle cure.

13.4 Dealing with Relapses

Few things are as frustrating as realizing that, despite all your efforts—improved diet, exercise, and self-care—the symptoms are suddenly back. Sometimes it's just a slight itch, sometimes a painful lump – but the feeling is always the same:

"Not again!"

Relapses are among the most discouraging moments in dealing with hemorrhoids because they shake your confidence in the progress you've made. But one thing should be clear: a relapse is not a personal failure.

Hemorrhoids are not like a simple wound that heals once and never returns. They are part of a complex condition involving diet, digestion, physical activity, stress levels, and individual tissue predispositions. And when the body's internal balance is thrown off – by travel, stress, an unhealthy phase, or just a "bad day" – old symptoms can flare up again.

What to Do When It Starts Again

First and foremost: stay calm. Panicking or throwing everything at the problem at once can overwhelm your body. A relapse is rarely a full setback to zero – it's usually just a temporary irritation. Often, a few simple measures are enough:

- **Eat lightly** to ease bowel movements
- **Drink plenty of fluids** to keep digestion moving
- **Use gentle hygiene** to avoid further irritation
- **Apply short-term topical** care, e.g., with a proven ointment
- **Reduce pressure** while sitting, e.g., with a seat cushion

In many cases, these steps can ease symptoms within a few days. The key is not to overreact, but to gently stabilize your routines.

Mindset Matters

A relapse doesn't just affect the body – it also hits your sense of self. Especially when you thought you had things "under control," a flare-up can feel like a major setback. Here, a calm mindset helps: relapses are part of the process, not the end of it.

Maybe you've been a little careless lately. Maybe you ignored your body's signals – or maybe it was just bad luck. The most important thing is: don't give up. Adjust and move forward. Those who respond calmly conserve energy and often return to a stable state more quickly.

Think Long-Term, Don't Fight Short-Term

Many people tend to question everything during a relapse: their diet, their treatment approach, their lifestyle. But often it's just a minor imbalance that's easy to correct. The goal is not to prevent relapses at all costs – but to develop a way of dealing with them that is neither panicked nor helpless.

People who take a long-term view don't see relapses as failures, but as part of a broader learning process. And that's what truly matters.

Surgery – Or Not Just Yet?

When symptoms persist for an extended period or when hemorrhoids have progressed to stage 3 or 4, the question quickly arises: should you consider surgery? Many specialists – particularly gastroenterologists or proctologists – will recommend surgery in such cases, often claiming that nothing else will help long-term.

But from my own experience, I would say:

Don't rush the decision.

Especially if you haven't yet tried more intensive alternative treatments, it can be worthwhile to give your body one more round of targeted support – for example, with remedies like MUCOKEHL D3, which act not just on the surface but on a deeper level. Or perhaps with a short, focused course of a more "radical" treatment like Ma Ying Long cream, which – though unusual – has in some cases led to a significant reduction of hemorrhoidal tissue.

Surgery is never a minor step. Even minimally invasive procedures like THD or traditional hemorrhoidectomy involve intervention in a highly sensitive area – with potential risks such as bleeding, pain, incontinence, or prolonged healing times.

Another critical consideration before surgery is whether the hemorrhoids might be part of a broader, chronic condition. Many people with hemorrhoids also suffer from digestive issues, irritable bowel syndrome, chronic stress, an imbalanced microbiome, or systemic connective tissue weakness.

In such cases, it often makes more sense to address not just the local symptoms, but also the underlying causes. Targeted gut restoration, strengthening the pelvic floor, reducing stress, or supplementing with supportive micronutrients can sometimes be more effective than a single surgical procedure.

Those who take the time to understand the bigger picture may not only avoid surgery – but also achieve a much higher level of overall health in the long run.

That's why you should honestly ask yourself before agreeing to surgery whether you've truly exhausted all gentler, regenerative options. Of course, there are situations where surgery is necessary and beneficial – for example, when symptoms severely impact daily life or complications arise.

But in many other cases, it's worth giving your body a few more weeks – with a deliberate attempt to find something that really works. If you then still opt for surgery, it will be with clarity – not out of pressure or frustration.

Chapter 14 – Movement, Body Awareness, and Everyday Habits

Anyone who thinks hemorrhoids can be treated purely on a physical level is missing a crucial part of the truth: how we move throughout the day, how we sit, work, breathe, or eat – all of this has a direct impact on the delicate vascular system in the rectal area. Many symptoms don't arise overnight but are the result of small, repeated strains, poor posture, or lack of movement.

The good news: the key to improvement often lies right there – in everyday life.

This chapter focuses on the practical levers that everyone can influence themselves. It's not about fitness programs or drastic lifestyle changes – but about mindful, often very simple adjustments that can bring noticeable relief.

In the first **section, 14.1**, we take a closer look at sitting posture and ergonomic work habits. Especially for those who spend a lot of time at a desk, small changes – like using a different chair, a hemorrhoid cushion, or taking conscious sitting breaks – can make a big difference.

The second **section, 14.2**, focuses on the often-overlooked pelvic floor. This muscle group is unconscious to many, yet essential for continence, circulation, and internal stability. I'll share simple exercises that are easy to integrate into daily life and provide lasting inner strength.

Section 14.3 explores the benefits of walking and moderate physical activity. Don't worry – this isn't about athletic performance. Even a short daily walk can work wonders – for circulation, digestion, and emotional balance.

To wrap things up, **section 14.4** invites you to explore the power of small rituals. Whether it's mindful sitting on the toilet, a short care routine, or five minutes of movement after a meal – it's often the unspectacular things that make the biggest difference over weeks and months.

This chapter is an invitation to stop seeing posture and movement as minor details – and instead to recognize them as part of the solution.

Those who gently change their everyday routines often change more than just their symptoms.

14.1 Proper Sitting and Ergonomic Work Habits

Many people today spend several hours a day sitting – at work, in the car, at the dining table, or on the couch. While this may seem harmless, it can be a crucial factor for those suffering from hemorrhoids. Prolonged sitting always means: increased pressure in the rectal area. Especially those who sit on hard chairs or in poor posture put strain on the sensitive vascular cushions – which may already be irritated or swollen. Over time, this leads to constant overstretching, worsening the condition or increasing the risk of relapse.

Sitting Posture: Small Changes, Big Impact

An upright posture with a slight forward tilt helps relieve pressure from the tailbone and reduces strain on the anal area. Ideally, the pelvis should be tilted slightly forward – not slumped backward, as often happens in soft armchairs or worn-out seats. The back should remain upright without becoming tense.

People who often "slouch" or sit in a rounded back position not only stress the spine but also the pelvic floor and the venous return system – which in turn can aggravate hemorrhoidal symptoms.

Making Smart Use of Ergonomic Aids

For many sufferers, a seat cushion with a tailbone cut-out (often referred to as a "hemorrhoid cushion") can offer immediate relief. It ensures that no direct pressure is placed on the sensitive area – which can be especially helpful during acute phases. Important: the cushion should not be too soft, as that leads to unstable posture again.

A height-adjustable chair, a flexible backrest, or a sit-stand desk setup can also make a big difference. Ergonomically optimizing your workspace often improves more than you expect – not just for your back, but also for the lower end of your digestive tract.

Microbreaks and Changing Positions

Besides posture itself, the rhythm of sitting is also crucial. Remaining in the same position for hours overloads specific areas of tissue. It's better to change positions regularly, stand up from time to time, do a few stretches, or simply take a short walk. Even just thirty seconds of movement per hour can improve venous circulation, relieve the pelvic floor, and boost blood flow. In many cases, this can ease minor relapses or pressure sensations without any medication at all.

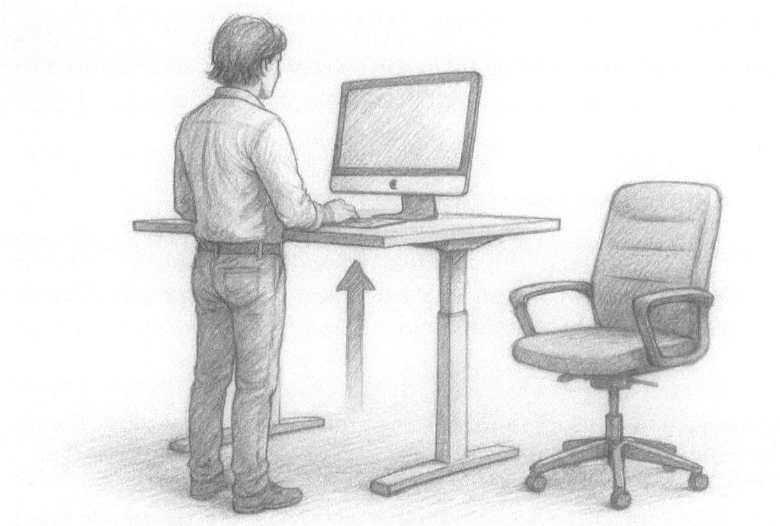

Conclusion: Creating the Foundation

Proper sitting isn't a cure-all – but it lays the groundwork for relief and healing. Those who sit a lot should not only focus on good posture but also develop small habits and tools to keep pressure as low as possible.

Because reducing pressure on the body over time gives it the chance to return to balance – gently, but effectively.

14.2 Exercises to Strengthen and Relieve the Pelvic Floor

Why the Pelvic Floor Is So Important

The pelvic floor is an invisible group of muscles that lies like a supportive net at the base of the torso. It holds the bladder, intestines, and internal organs in position and plays a direct role in continence, bowel function, and venous blood return. When it becomes weakened – through prolonged sitting, excess weight, constipation, or poor posture – the rectum loses its natural tension. The result: hemorrhoids can enlarge or return more easily.

The good news: the pelvic floor can be specifically trained – without equipment, without much effort, and often unnoticed in daily life. That's what makes it such a quiet but powerful key to greater stability and relief in the anal area.

Exercise 1: The Classic Contraction Exercise

Sit upright in a chair or stand with your feet hip-width apart. Inhale calmly – and as you exhale, consciously contract your pelvic floor, as if trying to stop the flow of urine or prevent a bowel movement. Hold this contraction for 3–5 seconds, then release.

Important: keep your buttocks and abdomen relaxed – only the pelvic floor should be active.

Repeat this 10–15 times in a row, ideally several times a day. You can do this in bed in the morning, in the car, at your desk, or on the couch in the evening – completely discreetly.

Exercise 2: The "Elevator Exercise"

Imagine your pelvic floor as an elevator with multiple floors. As you inhale, the elevator gently "descends." As you exhale, it slowly pulls back "up" – floor by floor.

This exercise helps build fine muscle control, not just basic tension, but nuanced awareness and movement.

Do this exercise slowly and with focus – it's especially useful when you want to center yourself or calm down.

Exercise 3: Relief While Lying Down

Lie on your back with your knees bent and your feet flat on the floor. Rest your hands gently on your lower abdomen. As you exhale, contract your pelvic floor; as you inhale, release. This position is especially relieving and ideal for beginners or during acute phases when sitting is uncomfortable.

You can also gently tilt your pelvis during this exercise – this promotes circulation and further reduces pressure in the rectal area.

Less Is More – But Be Consistent

Pelvic floor training isn't about intensity, but about regularity and mindfulness. Just two to three minutes a day are often enough – what matters is sticking with it. Even regular walks or standing upright with good posture support the pelvic floor and reduce strain during sitting or straining.

Those who commit to this muscle group are often surprised by how much strength, stability, and self-control can emerge from it – quite literally.

14.3 The Benefits of Walking and Moderate Movement

Hemorrhoids are not purely a "sitting problem" – but excessive sitting definitely worsens the symptoms. Conversely, this means: regular movement increases blood flow to the pelvic area, activates venous return, and stimulates bowel activity – three key factors for healing and preventing hemorrhoids.

This doesn't require a fitness program. On the contrary, many people find that gentle, moderate movement is far more effective than excessive ambition. Walking, casual cycling, or light yoga are more than enough to bring the body into a healthy rhythm. Circulation improves, digestion becomes more regular – and the pelvic floor is activated gently and naturally without being strained.

Walking: The Underestimated Healing Impulse

A daily walk – even just 20 to 30 minutes – can work wonders. It releases tension, calms the mind, and helps resolve pelvic congestion caused by prolonged sitting. A brisk yet relaxed pace is particularly beneficial – ideally in nature, without a phone, without distractions. Many people notice that after a walk, their lower abdomen feels lighter, and the anal area less pressured.

Walking is also a great way to reduce stress, which in turn supports gut health and mucosal regeneration through hormonal processes. Making walking a daily ritual not only improves physical health – it also strengthens emotional stability.

No Overexertion – But Regularity

What should be avoided are excessive physical stresses like heavy lifting, intense abdominal workouts, or high-pressure activities (such as weightlifting or long-distance running on hard surfaces). These can worsen symptoms or trigger relapses. The body doesn't need force – it needs gentle, consistent activation.

The goal is not to exhaust yourself but to keep moving. Even small doses of daily activity – taking the stairs instead of the elevator, running errands on foot, or a short walk after meals – can add up over time to make a real difference in your health.

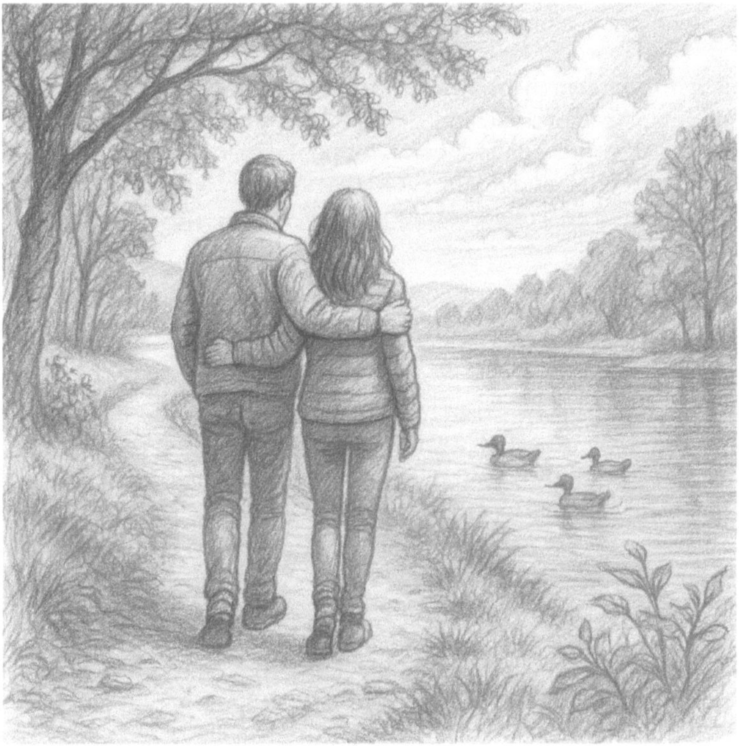

Conclusion: Movement as a Core Attitude

Movement isn't an optional extra you "should also do" – it's a foundational part of recovery. Those who move regularly help their body release pressure, support healing processes, and prevent relapses. And the best part: it doesn't require anything complicated. A good pair of shoes and a bit of time are all you need. Your body will do the rest – if you let it.

14.4 Small Rituals, Big Impact

Healing comes through repetition. When dealing with hemorrhoids, most people first think of medications, ointments, or special treatments. What's often overlooked: it's the small things you do regularly that have the greatest impact. It's not the spectacular interventions, but the quiet, everyday habits that determine whether healing occurs – or symptoms return.

A glass of warm water in the morning, a short walk after a meal, a few minutes of sitting upright instead of slouching – all of this may seem insignificant, but over time, it creates an entirely different environment within the body. Rituals provide the body with structure and rhythm. And that's exactly what disrupted processes – such as an irritated anal region or sluggish digestion – need in order to recover sustainably.

Three Everyday Examples

The Conscious Toilet Visit: Instead of rushing or straining, take a calm moment – ideally at the same time each day. Sitting in a relaxed posture without pressing (possibly with feet slightly elevated) reduces pressure on the rectum and helps prevent irritation. A simple footstool can work wonders here.

The Daily Care Ritual: After showering or a bowel movement, take a brief pause and gently treat the anal area with a soothing remedy – perhaps a trusted ointment or a bit of olive oil. It only takes 30 seconds, but the effect adds up. More importantly, it sends a signal to your body: You are being taken seriously.

Movement After Meals: A short walk – even just five minutes – boosts circulation and supports bowel activity. Making this a habit after lunch or dinner can significantly improve digestion without the need for additional aids.

The Body Loves Rhythm

Many complaints arise from inconsistency and stress. When everything is constantly changing – mealtimes, sleep patterns, physical activity, mental load – the body loses its sense of balance. Small rituals create stability – not as rigid rules, but as gentle acts of self-care. Those who grant themselves a few fixed "anchor points" during the day relieve pressure – both mentally and physically.

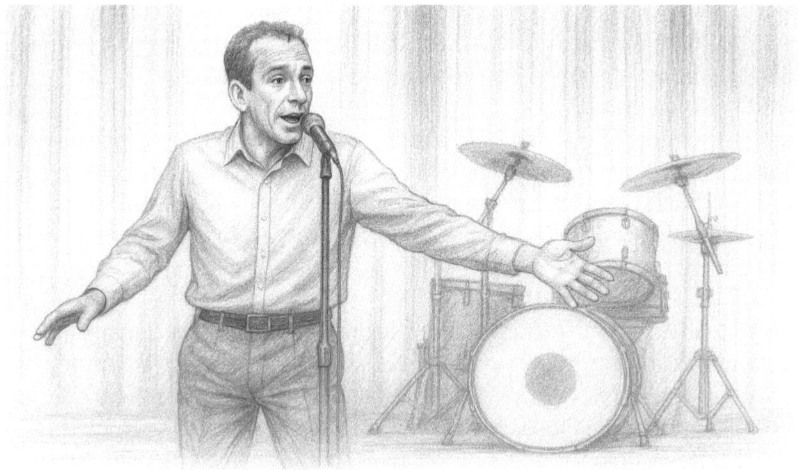

You've got to feel the groove...

Conclusion: Low Effort, High Impact

Most people underestimate how much influence they have on their own health through small daily habits. You don't have to change everything – starting with just one or two rituals is enough. Giving your body a little conscious attention each day not only strengthens your physical health but also builds confidence:

I can help myself.

And that's often the first step toward lasting improvement.

Chapter 15 – The Mental Aspect: Stress, Shame, and Body Awareness

Many people suffering from hemorrhoids look for the cause solely in the physical realm: poor diet, lack of exercise, too much sitting. And yes – all of that plays a role, no question. But the body is not an isolated system. It reacts to what we think, feel, expect, or suppress. And the rectal area, in particular, is one of the places where inner tension tends to show up quickly – through pressure sensations, cramps, burning, or pain.

This chapter shifts the focus to the mental and emotional level: the interplay between the nervous system, perception, and body posture.

Section 15.1 explores how psychological pressure can intensify physical symptoms. Chronic stress, inner restlessness, or emotional tension often manifest in places you'd least expect – in the gut, the pelvic floor, or the anal region. Understanding this connection reveals that sometimes, relaxation helps more than any ointment.

Section 15.2 addresses the journey from suppression to active engagement. Hemorrhoids are a topic many prefer to avoid – out of shame, discomfort, or insecurity. But this very avoidance often prevents healing. Those who dare to confront the issue openly lose the fear – and regain a sense of agency. This section also shows how tools like AI – such as ChatGPT – can be used for guided self-reflection, helping to uncover hidden causes and understand oneself more deeply.

Section 15.3 shines a light on a rarely discussed but powerful substance: lithium as nourishment for the brain. In small doses, lithium can have a calming effect on the nervous system, ease emotional tension, and reduce chronic tightness. For many, it is the missing puzzle piece that allows them to find inner calm – and give the body space to regenerate.

Finally, **section 15.4** addresses what may be the hardest – but most transformative – step: self-acceptance and an open view of one's own body. Healing is not possible when we reject ourselves. True change begins when we are willing to meet ourselves with compassion and respect – even in the uncomfortable or shame-filled parts. Not through struggle – but through acceptance.

15.1 How Psychological Pressure Intensifies Physical Symptoms

Many people initially perceive physical complaints like hemorrhoids as purely mechanical: too much sitting, too little movement, poor diet. And yes – that's true, but only partly. What is often overlooked: psychological pressure, chronic stress, and suppressed emotions also manifest in the body. Not in some abstract way – but in very real, tangible, painful ways.

The rectal area is especially sensitive. It belongs to those parts of the body we are least aware of – and often associate most strongly with shame, control, and tension. Those who constantly push themselves in daily life, never take breaks, or live in a state of inner pressure, unknowingly transfer that tension to the muscles of the pelvic floor, lower abdomen, and around the anus. Chronic tension reduces blood flow, increases pressure sensations, and disrupts the natural rhythm of digestion. And this is exactly where hemorrhoids can develop – or repeatedly flare up.

Control, Pressure, Avoidance

Sensitive or high-achieving individuals in particular tend to suppress discomfort, hide what's bothering them, and "push through." But this very behavior leads the body to speak in its own way. If stress isn't expressed, it's swallowed – or in this case: pressed.

A constant tightness builds in the abdomen, an unconscious holding – even during bowel movements.

Defecation becomes something to get over with as quickly as possible. People sit down tense, strain, want to be done – and overlook the fact that they're working against the natural process.

The body responds with symptoms: hemorrhoids, pressure, irritation.

Not because it's "sick" – but because it wants to send a signal:

"Stop. This isn't working."

The First Step: Face It Instead of Suppressing It

Recognizing this connection is the first step out of the purely symptom-based approach. It's not about over-psychologizing everything, but understanding: body and mind are not opposites – they are one system.

And when that system is overloaded, the answer isn't to add more pressure – but to relieve it.

This might mean allowing yourself breaks. Letting feelings arise. Stopping the habit of overburdening yourself. Or very practically: taking time for your bowel movements, instead of rushing through them as a bothersome task.

Those who let go emotionally often find it easier to let go physically as well – and that, for many people with hemorrhoids, is the true turning point.

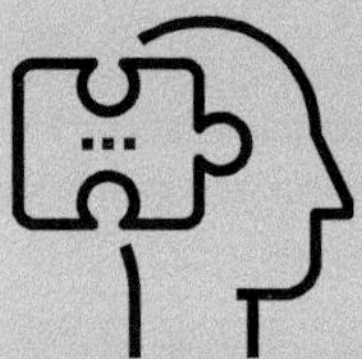

Did You Know…?

There is a connection between gut health and mental well-being. The so-called gut-brain axis is directly linked via nerve pathways – an imbalance in the gut can affect mood, concentration, and energy levels.

15.2 From Suppression to Active Engagement

Many people who suffer from hemorrhoids gradually develop an inner distance from their bodies – especially from the area "down there." The symptoms are unpleasant, the region is associated with shame, and there's a strong hope that "it will just go away." So the issue gets ignored, postponed, suppressed. People don't want to deal with it – and certainly not talk about it.

The problem is: what we suppress doesn't disappear.

It builds up – not just mentally, but physically. The anal area is a place where both physical and emotional tension can accumulate quickly. Those who feel overwhelmed, unseen, or who neglect their own needs often don't notice it in their mood – but through itching, pressure, or burning sensations. The body finds a way to be heard.

The Turning Point: Taking Responsibility

Suppression only works until the body becomes so loud that you can't ignore it anymore. But this is also where the opportunity lies: those who are willing to face it can begin to shift the dynamic. Not instantly, not with a single step – but with a clear decision:

I'm going to face this. I want to know what's going on. And I'm going to take care of it.

This mindset changes everything. Suddenly it's no longer just about eliminating a symptom – but about seeing your body as an ally. Not as an enemy that gets in the way, but as a messenger saying,

"Something's not right. And you can do something about it."

Active engagement often starts with something simple: reading up on the topic. Taking a pelvic floor class. Paying more attention to your diet. Or no longer seeing bowel movements as a nuisance, but as a small act of self-care. The more you engage with the topic, the less shame remains – and the more confidently you'll handle it.

From Suffering to a Learning Process

Hemorrhoids are not a personal failure. But they can be a sign of imbalance – physical, emotional, or lifestyle-related. Recognizing this takes away the feeling of helplessness. And those who are willing to learn from it regain a sense of self-respect. What once felt like a burden becomes an opportunity for change. Not because you have to – but because you want to. Because you realize: I'm allowed to take care of myself. And that is often the first step toward true healing.

Using AI for Self-Reflection

Sometimes it's hard to start a conversation with yourself. You feel that something's wrong – physically or emotionally – but your thoughts keep circling, staying on the surface, or are so unclear you don't know where to begin. This is exactly where artificial intelligence – especially language models like ChatGPT – can offer surprisingly effective support.

Instead of getting lost in your own head, you can start talking to the AI – in writing or via voice message, depending on the app or device.

It's not about getting a diagnosis or replacing therapy.

It's about organizing your thoughts, seeing things more clearly, and making connections that might otherwise stay hidden.

You can start simply:

- *"I'm feeling that pressure again – what could be causing it?"*
- *"I notice I'm often tense on the toilet – could that be related to stress?"*
- *"How can I treat my body more mindfully without having to change everything at once?"*

The AI doesn't respond like an all-knowing therapist, but more like an attentive conversation partner – helping you structure your thoughts, ask better questions, and make connections. Especially with shame-related or sensitive topics – like hemorrhoids or body issues – talking to an AI can offer a low-threshold, safe way to honestly engage with yourself.

It becomes especially powerful when done regularly. Some people write a few lines every morning, others send themselves voice notes that are transcribed and answered by the app. This creates a dialogue that's not just analytical but can also bring emotional relief. It's like learning to connect with yourself – with a calm, non-judgmental voice on the other side that never interrupts.

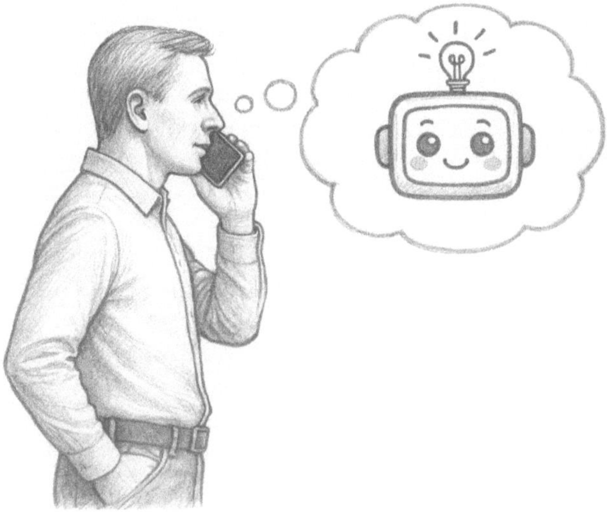

Especially for psychosomatic conditions like hemorrhoids – where physical symptoms often have an emotional background – this kind of reflection can help uncover the underlying dynamics.

Suddenly you realize when your body is reacting, what situations create pressure, and where old patterns are still active. And from that awareness, change becomes possible – not through force, but through understanding.

Those who discover this path for themselves may come to see: Conversations with AI aren't a substitute for real human connection – but they can be a reliable mirror, a quiet companion on the journey toward deeper self-awareness.

And sometimes, that's the beginning of a new relationship with yourself – even, or especially, when the topic seems as trivial as hemorrhoids.

15.3 Lithium as Nutrition for the Brain

An Underrated Trace Element: In public perception, lithium is almost exclusively known as a medication for severe psychiatric conditions – such as the treatment of manic episodes or depression. What many people don't know: lithium occurs naturally in the environment – in drinking water, plants, and soil – and it serves important functions in the body, even in very small amounts.

At low doses – far below the therapeutic levels used in psychiatry – lithium has neuroprotective, anti-inflammatory, and mood-stabilizing effects. Studies have shown that in regions with slightly higher lithium levels in the drinking water, both suicide rates and general stress levels are lower. Additionally, concentration, emotional balance, and impulse control appear to be more stable when lithium intake is adequate.

Calming the Nervous System – Felt Throughout the Body

What does this have to do with hemorrhoids? Much more than you might think at first. Many of the symptoms around the anal area aren't just local in origin – they're systemic, caused by chronic tension, inner restlessness, or suppressed stress. The pelvic floor is a sensitive area that responds strongly to the autonomic nervous system.

Those who are constantly tense also "hold on" physically – and this often leads to constipation, straining during bowel movements, and ultimately irritation of the hemorrhoidal cushions.

Lithium can help precisely at this level. It regulates the central nervous system, stabilizes signal transmission in the brain, and reduces overactive stress patterns. Many people report that taking microdoses of lithium (e.g., lithium orotate at 1–5 mg per day) brings a sense of inner calm they hadn't experienced before – not a "sedated" feeling, but a gentle relaxation of the inner system.

And this relaxation often extends to the body: muscle tension eases, breathing becomes deeper and calmer, and digestion improves.

A Tool for Regulation – Not for Numbing

It's important to understand: this is not about high-dose therapy or prescription medications, but about the mindful use of natural microdoses – similar to the levels found in certain mineral waters.

Those who suffer from ongoing restlessness, tension, or psychosomatic symptoms may benefit from low-dose lithium as a gentle form of support – comparable to magnesium, but working on a deeper neurological level.

Of course, lithium is not a miracle cure. But it can be a valuable tool in managing stress-related conditions – especially when the body won't let go, even though the mind wants to.

For some, it may be the missing piece to regaining enough balance for healing to even begin.

Safety and Use

Anyone considering lithium as a dietary supplement should ensure the dosage is low (e.g., lithium orotate with 1 to 5 mg of elemental lithium per day) and consult a healthcare provider if unsure. These supplements are available over the counter and are approved as dietary supplements in many countries. It's important to monitor the effects mindfully – and not to exceed the recommended dosage. The goal is not sedation, but a gentle return to inner stability.

In Western Europe, lithium orotate is not officially approved as a dietary supplement, but it can still be obtained – for example, as a liquid form via online platforms such as Amazon.

15.4 Self-Acceptance and a New Perspective on Your Body

Your body is not the enemy: Those who suffer from hemorrhoids over a longer period often develop a strained relationship with their body – especially with the area where the symptoms occur. The anal region is already a taboo topic, and when pain, bleeding, or itching appear repeatedly, a sense of alienation or rejection can quickly follow. Many would prefer to ignore "down there" – or fix it, as if it were a broken part.

But this attitude often creates the opposite of what is hoped for: more tension, more pressure, more shame. Self-rejection leads to chronic stress – and that stress directly affects the nervous system, muscles, and pain perception.

Stop Avoiding Yourself

An important step toward healing is learning to look at your body with openness and kindness – including the uncomfortable or unloved parts. That doesn't mean sugarcoating the problem or pretending the symptoms "aren't so bad." It means acknowledging what is – and relating to it.

A simple start can be to stop seeing the affected area as merely functional and instead as part of a whole – part of you.

If your arm were sore, you'd naturally care for it. So why not treat the anal area with the same matter-of-fact attention? Not with disgust, but with respect.

Your body isn't foreign – it is you.

Let Go of Shame, Preserve Your Dignity

Many people with hemorrhoids experience a deep, often hard-to-define sense of shame. It's not just the fear of smell or bleeding – it's a feeling that "something is wrong" with them as a person. But shame isolates. And isolation intensifies suffering. That's why it's so important not to accept this shame as truth, but to recognize it for what it is: a learned response that can be questioned.

Self-acceptance means seeing yourself not only in the light, but also in the shadow – and embracing both.

The body is a process, not a finished product. Everyone has weak spots, scars, quirks. That doesn't make us less worthy – it makes us human.

Healing Begins with Acceptance

Many people report that their symptoms improved when they stopped fighting against them – and instead began truly caring for themselves. Not just externally, but internally.

Those who accept themselves – including their symptoms – create the space in which regeneration becomes possible.

Not through force, but through compassion.

Because in the end, with hemorrhoids – as with many chronic conditions – it's not only about what's happening in the tissue.

It's about what's happening between you and your body.

And when that dialogue becomes more honest, healing can sometimes begin exactly where you had given up hope.

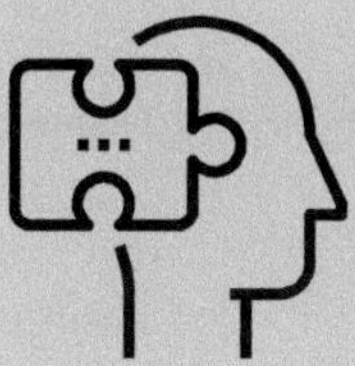

Did You Know…?

Lithium is not only found in medications – it is also a natural component of certain medicinal waters. One of the most well-known is Staatl. Fachingen, but waters like Adelheidquelle or Heppinger also contain notable amounts in some cases.

Chapter 16 – My Personal Conclusion

After more than ten years with hemorrhoids – including relapses, surgeries, hope, disappointment, and an entirely new perspective on my body – it's time for a personal conclusion. Not a medical summary, but an honest reflection:

What worked? What didn't? And what have I learned from it?

This chapter is not meant to be a guide, but an invitation to reflect. Because in the end, every journey is individual – but certain patterns can become clear if you look closely.

This final chapter looks back on what's behind me, but it also looks forward – for you as a reader, and for anyone dealing with similar issues.

In **section 16.1**, I share my personal journey: two failed surgeries, a period of truly intense symptoms – and then a gradual improvement that didn't come from another medical intervention, but from a shift in perspective. The realization that the issue wasn't just in the anal area – it required a holistic approach.

Section 16.2 explores why that holistic view is so essential. The body is not a mechanical system with interchangeable parts – it's a sensitive, interconnected organism. If you treat only what's visible, you often miss what's most important. And those who are open to connections – between posture, stress, the nervous system, and internal experience – sometimes find completely new paths toward relief.

And in the final section 16.3, I offer a personal appeal:

More openness, less shame. Hemorrhoids are not a weakness. They are a signal. And it's worth listening to that signal – not with fear, but with curiosity. Not with guilt, but with self-respect.

This chapter doesn't end the book with a "solution," but with a different point of view:

You are allowed to trust your body.

And you are allowed to **take your time getting to know it** – fully, deeply, and without judgment.

16.1 A Look Back at More Than Ten Years with Hemorrhoids

Two Surgeries, Many Insights –

and a New Relationship with My Body

The Beginning: The Hope for a Clear Solution

When the symptoms first began, my initial reaction was: There must be something that can fix this.

Like many others, I started with ointments, home remedies, and well-meaning advice – all without lasting success. Eventually, things progressed to the point where the hemorrhoids weren't just annoying – they became severe. At times, the swollen tissue was the size of a cherry, sometimes even larger, and I had to push it back in with two or three fingers just to sit or walk normally. It wasn't just physically unpleasant – it was mentally exhausting.

Surgery seemed like the obvious next step.

I took that step – twice.

But in hindsight, it wasn't the solution I had hoped for. The first operation brought only brief relief. The second – supposedly done "the right way" – turned out to be a complete failure. And with it came the realization:

Maybe this isn't the path my body needs.

Disappointment – and Then a New Perspective

It was deeply frustrating to still be in pain after two surgeries. But it also marked a turning point. I began to understand that my hemorrhoids weren't just a local issue – but part of a broader, more complex system.

The real shift didn't come from another medical appointment, but from treating my CMD (craniomandibular dysfunction). During the past three years of holistic treatment, my hemorrhoids significantly improved – without any further surgery, without new creams, without drastic interventions.

That, to me, was proof:

The body is a system.

And when something falls out of balance in one area, it can show up in a completely different place.

I learned to look more closely, to observe what was happening to me – not just in terms of symptoms, but the bigger picture. And I became more cautious. More cautious with snap decisions. More cautious with the thought:

"This needs to go – now."

Surgery: Not Wrong by Default – But Often Too Soon

Today, I'm convinced that surgery isn't inherently bad – but it should truly be the last resort. I wish I had taken more time back then, had more trust in my body, and more holistic support. Looking back, I don't believe I'd be worse off today had I skipped the surgeries. In fact, I might have spared myself a lot – scars, fear, and a feeling of losing control. That doesn't mean I regret the past.
But I've learned from it:

Not everything that's technically possible is the right choice. Sometimes, what's needed isn't more intervention – but more insight.

Today: Accepted, Stable – and Largely Symptom-Free

Today I live with my hemorrhoids in a condition I would almost call unproblematic. They've become much smaller, often barely noticeable, and I can live with them very well – without surgery, without acute interventions.

I've learned to understand and care for my body differently. I listen more closely, respond earlier, and have become more patient with myself.

And most importantly: I would never rush into surgery again. I now know the body can find its own way – sometimes surprising, sometimes slow – to restore balance.

You just have to give it the chance.

16.2 Why a Holistic Perspective Is Essential

Symptoms are not disruptions – they are signals.

In conventional medicine, it's common to treat a problem exactly where it appears. If hemorrhoids are painful, then the treatment focuses on the rectal area. Ointments, suppositories, surgeries – all target the local zone of symptoms.

But this tunnel vision is often the reason why the complaints don't improve in the long run. What appears on the surface to be a purely mechanical or inflammatory issue is often part of a much broader imbalance.

The human body does not function in isolation. Muscles, the nervous system, digestion, hormonal balance, and the psyche – everything is interconnected. When something is chronically "stuck" in one area, it's worth looking at the surrounding systems.

Especially in the case of hemorrhoids, it often becomes clear: those who treat only the visible symptoms tend to overlook the root causes – which may lie somewhere entirely different.

Everything Is Connected

There are many examples of this. Tension in the jaw (CMD) can affect the entire posture chain – all the way to the pelvic floor. Chronic stress alters gut flora and changes how pain is perceived. Unconscious tension in the abdomen can lead to shallow breathing – which in turn activates the nervous system and slows down digestion. And those who internally reject themselves will rarely find peace in their body.

In my own case – where symptoms improved significantly during CMD treatment – this became very clear:

The hemorrhoids were not an isolated problem, but an expression of a deeper imbalance. That doesn't mean everything has to be psychologized. But it does mean:

Those who take a holistic view will see more – and go further.

A New Relationship with the Body

A holistic perspective also means becoming mindful, thinking in terms of root causes, and giving the body a voice again. It's not about treating everything at once – but about recognizing relationships:

between posture and circulation, between emotions and physical tension, between diet and inflammation.

Often, it's enough to make a conscious change in just one or two areas – and the system begins to regulate itself. This doesn't require a radical lifestyle shift, but rather a stable foundation of understanding, patience, and awareness. The body has a remarkable ability to heal itself – but it needs the right conditions.

From Repair to Regeneration

The difference is profound:

Those who aim to repair focus on symptoms. Those who support regeneration guide the process. In the first case, the goal is to quickly "function" again. In the second, healing is allowed to unfold – even if it takes longer.

A holistic perspective doesn't mean being esoteric. It simply means: not just treating what's visible, but also understanding what's invisible –

- the nervous system,
- emotional patterns,
- movement habits,
- inner resistance.

Once you've experienced it – for example, the connection between CMD treatment and the improvement of hemorrhoids – you begin to see:

The body is intelligent.

And when we learn to listen, it often tells us exactly what it needs.

16.3 A Call for More Openness, Less Shame

What you refuse to see can still heal – if you're willing to look.

You're Not Alone

Hemorrhoids are a taboo topic. Nearly every second person develops them at some point in life – but hardly anyone talks about them openly. Instead, people suffer in silence, suppress the issue, hope it will go away. Many feel alone, helpless, or even ashamed.

That's why it's so important to break the silence – and this book ends deliberately with a call:

Don't be afraid of the topic. And especially, don't be afraid of yourself.

If you've read this book, then you've already taken the brave step of confronting a topic that many would rather avoid. And that alone is a first step toward healing. Not every solution is surgical. Not every path goes through conventional medicine.

And above all: **Not everything that's uncomfortable has to stay that way forever.**

A Broader Perspective Can Change Everything

What helps many people with hemorrhoids isn't another ointment or a third suppository – but a shift in perspective. Maybe it's not just a problem at the anus. Maybe it's part of a more complex pattern: posture, nervous system, body alignment, lifestyle. And that's why it can sometimes be more helpful not to seek out yet another proctologist – but to look elsewhere.

A holistic dentist, an experienced osteopath, a thoughtful orthopedic specialist – people who understand the connections between posture, muscle chains, stress, and internal tension – may be able to contribute more than expected.Especially when traditional approaches haven't brought relief, it's worth having the courage to try something new.

The body is a system – and the solution is not always where the symptom appears.

A Body That Wants to Be Seen

What this path needs most is openness and patience. Many chronic conditions don't disappear with a single intervention – but they do change when we begin to take them seriously, without letting them define us.

Healing is not a promise – but a process.

And that process often doesn't begin with surgery – but with an honest question to yourself:

What do I really need?

Those who are willing to ask that question – without fear, without shame, but with curiosity – will eventually find a path.

Not a perfect one. Not an instant one. But a real one.

In Closing: You're Allowed to Take Your Time

If there's one thing you take from this book, let it be this:

You're allowed to take your time.

You don't have to "get rid of" anything. You don't have to decide right away. And you are not broken just because you're dealing with a problem others don't want to see.

Your body is a wise system. And if you learn to listen to it, over time it will show you what truly helps.

More openness. Less shame. More trust. Less pressure.

That's not medical advice – it's an invitation:

To treat yourself with a little more warmth and respect.

And maybe that's the best place to begin.

Appendix & Resources

AI as a Tool for Self-Awareness

In the previous chapters, the focus was often on the body – on ointments, movement, nutrition, stress, and internal tension. But ultimately, all of this leads to one central question: How well am I in touch with myself? Many health issues don't just arise from external circumstances, but from a lack of inner awareness. And this is precisely where modern technology can play a surprisingly helpful role.

Artificial intelligence – especially in the form of language models like ChatGPT – is far more than just a technical gimmick. When used mindfully, it can serve as a guide, a partner in reflection, and a quiet companion on the journey toward deeper self-awareness. No judgment, no time pressure, no shame.

In this chapter, I'll show you how to make use of this opportunity – in a practical, everyday-friendly way that suits your personal style.

In the first section, we explore why self-reflection is often so difficult – and how AI can help create inner clarity. Precisely because it doesn't judge or interrupt, AI can become an unusual but very helpful conversation partner.

In the second section, you'll discover three everyday scenarios that illustrate how such conversations might look – from pressure sensations at your desk, to physical tension on the toilet, to dealing with relapses. You'll get examples of phrasing and learn how to recognize whether you're avoiding yourself – or truly meeting yourself.

In the third section, I'll show you how to establish a simple reflection routine using short voice messages or daily five-minute sessions. The advantage over a traditional journal lies in the structured, dialog-based format – and in the fact that you're speaking to someone who's actually "there."

Finally, the forth section explores the limits and possibilities: What can AI really do – and what can't it? Where does it serve as a mirror, and where might it become a dead end? And what do you need to bring to the table for it to truly help?

This chapter is not a tech promotion – it's an invitation:

To begin a new kind of conversation with yourself. Open, honest – and with a counterpart who never gets tired of listening.

Why Self-Reflection Is So Difficult – and How AI Can Help

Observing oneself sounds easy – but it's not. Most of us know surprisingly little about what's really going on inside us. We notice physical discomfort, may realize we're irritable or feeling off, but the exact connection often remains vague.

The reason is simple: we live within ourselves. And that's precisely what makes objective self-awareness so hard.

Our perception is shaped by expectations, self-protection, habits – and often by the fear of discovering something unpleasant. Many thoughts run automatically, many emotions are instinctively suppressed. As a result, physical tension, recurring symptoms or chronic ailments emerge – without us being fully aware of the inner cause.

Especially with issues like hemorrhoids – which are associated with shame, withdrawal, or physical overwhelm – it's hard to have an open conversation with oneself. We avoid it. Or we think too quickly that we've "already figured it out." In doing so, we often miss the crucial insight:

It's not knowledge that heals – it's the genuine, repeated encounter with ourselves.

The Benefit of a Dialogic Counterpart

Self-reflection becomes easier when there's a counterpart.

Someone who listens, asks questions, mirrors your thoughts – or simply is there without judgment. A good conversation partner can provide structure, illuminate blind spots, or offer new perspectives – all without making you feel attacked.

But not everyone has such a person in their daily life. And even if you do: some topics are too intimate, too laden with shame, or too unclear to share. This is where an artificial intelligence like ChatGPT can play a surprisingly helpful role – not as a replacement for therapy, but as a patient, structured counterpart.

In written dialogue – or even spoken input via an app – a space suddenly opens up. You can express what moves you, without being interrupted. You receive questions that encourage reflection but don't pressure you. And you stay entirely with yourself – without feeling the need to explain or justify.

AI as a Structured, Nonjudgmental Instance

What makes AI so unique isn't just its availability – it's its posture.

It doesn't judge. It doesn't interrupt. It doesn't get annoyed, shrug, or feel overwhelmed. That makes it a neutral mirror in which you can encounter yourself anew.

ChatGPT is not emotional – but it is responsive. It can understand what you express, offer impulses, help sort your thoughts, identify patterns – and sometimes ask just the right question to untangle a crucial knot.

Not because it "knows who you are," but because it stays open, responds kindly, and helps you bring clarity to things you might not grasp on your own.

Especially with psychosomatic issues like hemorrhoids – where emotions, body perception, and lifestyle are closely interwoven – this kind of AI-supported self-reflection can be a real tool.

Not dramatic. Not "spiritual."

Simply and effectively: a quiet dialogue that helps you understand yourself better.

Conversation Examples with ChatGPT – From Symptom to Insight

How a simple exchange can lead to new clarity

Three concrete everyday scenes

1st Scene: There's pressure – and you don't know why

You've been sitting at your desk for two hours. Suddenly, you feel that pressure again. Nothing dramatic, but enough to make you tense up inside. You notice yourself getting annoyed – with your body, with yourself. In the past, you would've just ignored it or quickly applied some ointment.

Today, you open ChatGPT and write:

"I'm feeling that pressure in my anus again. It often happens when I work for a long time. Can you help me understand what's behind it?"

The AI might respond with a follow-up question:

"What exactly does the pressure feel like? And what happens in your body when you notice it?"

And suddenly you realize: it's not just physical. It's a kind of inner constriction. Maybe because you're doing something that's too much for you right now. Or because you've been putting pressure on yourself. Through the conversation, you begin to see not just the symptom – but the pattern.

2nd Scene: On the toilet – everything is tense again

You're sitting on the toilet. It's taking time. You're not straining, but you feel it: nothing's moving. Everything is tight. And there it is again, that old voice in your head: "You're not functioning."

Instead of getting frustrated, you speak it out loud – as a short voice-to-text input:

"I'm sitting on the toilet right now and I'm completely tense. Nothing's happening. What could be behind this?"

The AI responds calmly, maybe something like:

"Do you feel like you're holding something back – not just physically, but emotionally too?"

That simple question can open something. Maybe your thoughts were still tied up in a difficult conversation. Maybe you haven't really "let go" yet, because you're still feeling tense inside. And suddenly, a blocked bowel movement becomes a deeper question:

What else am I holding onto – inside me?

3rd Scene: A relapse – and the old helplessness

After weeks of improvement, suddenly: blood, pressure, fear. The hemorrhoids are back. You feel helpless. Frustrated. A setback. Powerless. You open the app, hesitate – and type:

"I just had another relapse. I thought I had it under control. Why is this hitting me so hard?"

The answer might be:

"What do you associate with the relapse – just the physical symptoms, or also a sense of having failed?"

And you realize: it's not really about the tissue. It's about the feeling of not making progress. Not being good enough. And the conversation with the AI becomes an invitation – to be gentler with yourself.

Example questions to get started

If you want to talk with ChatGPT, you don't need to know anything – just be willing to write honestly. Here are some questions you might try:

- *"What might my body be trying to tell me right now?"*
- *"Why is it so hard for me to truly relax?"*
- *"I feel pressure inside – where could that be coming from?"*

- *"How can I learn to listen better to my body?"*
- *"I'm afraid of having a relapse – how can I deal with that?"*
- *"I feel ashamed about my symptoms – what might be behind that?"*

The AI won't give perfect answers. But it will ask the right counter-questions – and that's often enough to shift your perspective.

How to tell if you're avoiding yourself – or being honest

Real self-reflection begins where things start to feel uncomfortable. If you notice yourself dodging the AI's questions so you don't have to look at yourself, that's a good sign:

You've reached the point where things get interesting.

Typical avoidance tactics include:

"I already know all this."

"This won't help."

"This is too exhausting right now."

But if you write what's really going on inside you – even if it feels messy or embarrassing – you'll notice that the conversation holds you. And suddenly, it's not about AI anymore – it's about you.

Self-reflection isn't a project for perfect people. It's a tool for real ones.

And AI can be a mirror – one that doesn't judge, doesn't look away, and never tires of staying in dialogue with you.

Voice Messages, Daily Routines & Journaling with AI

A new way to listen to yourself – through digital means

How to use voice-to-text to turn AI into a listener

Sometimes your head is full of thoughts – but the moment you try to sit down and write, everything gets blocked. Too exhausting, too complicated, too vague. This is exactly where the combination of spoken language and artificial intelligence can offer a surprisingly simple and effective entry into self-reflection.

Modern AI applications like ChatGPT can be used not just via keyboard, but also through voice. In the smartphone app, you can simply speak your thoughts out loud, the text is transcribed automatically – and the AI responds like in a normal chat.

This form of interaction is especially helpful when you're in the middle of an emotional moment: while walking, sitting on the couch, driving, or right after a stressful situation.

You don't need perfect wording. Just say what's going on inside you – just as you would tell someone who truly listens. The AI becomes your neutral, never-annoyed conversation partner, who listens, asks follow-up questions, or simply organizes what you've said.

Daily 5-minute sessions: Questions, prompts, pattern recognition

It's especially helpful to establish a short daily routine – for example, in the morning after waking up or at night before going to bed. Just five minutes are enough to become more aware of your day, recognize patterns, or sense emotional tension early.

An example of a daily session might look like this:

You speak:

"Today was a good day – but I always feel this pressure after lunch. It annoys me because I actually think I'm doing everything right."

The AI replies:

"Was there anything today that weighed on you emotionally – maybe not directly related to food, but more on a psychological level?"

You realize:

"That's true. I had a conversation with my boss that stressed me more than I thought."

This creates a mini-dialogue that requires no big explanations – yet still brings new insights. And if you do this regularly, over time you'll begin to notice recurring patterns: repeated triggers, internal tensions, small shifts in how you feel.

The chat with AI becomes a kind of digital mirror ritual – always available, never overwhelming.

Reflection advantages compared to a traditional journal

A classic diary has its place – but it remains one-sided. You write in it, but you don't get any feedback. No questions, no prompts. AI changes that: it gives you a second perspective. And sometimes, it's precisely that follow-up question that leads you to a thought that would never have entered your awareness otherwise.

Another benefit: you don't have to push yourself to write perfectly. No "I don't know how to start." No blank pages. You can speak, write, shorten, stumble, jump around – the AI follows you. And it helps you find the red thread, even when you think you've lost it.

Especially with bodily issues, where emotion, shame, helplessness, and hope are tightly intertwined, this form of guided reflection with a digital counterpart can be liberating. Not as a replacement for human connection – but as a supplement that's available around the clock and helps you take yourself seriously.

Limits & Possibilities – and What Not to Expect

Between Tool and Companion: How AI Can Truly Help

AI is no replacement for therapy

As helpful as artificial intelligence can be – it has clear limitations. It can listen, ask questions, organize your thoughts, and offer impulses. But it is not a therapist, not a human being, and not a feeling entity. It won't see your facial expressions, interpret your tone of voice, or sense your silence. And most importantly: it doesn't know your life context – only what you choose to share.

If you are struggling with deep psychological burdens, if trauma, depression, or anxiety significantly affect your life, an exchange with AI is not enough. In such cases, it's important to seek professional help – from real people trained to work with depth, empathy, and therapeutic responsibility.

AI is not a crisis responder. It is no substitute for real human connection. But it can be a starting point – or a supportive resource that finds its place between therapy sessions, during long periods of reflection, or as a daily partner for self-inquiry.

AI can be a reliable, structured mirror

What AI can offer – and what many people lack in daily life – is a constant, calm form of attention. AI won't interrupt you. It won't judge you. It never loses patience. And it doesn't ask questions out of curiosity – but to help you gain clarity.

In doing so, it becomes a kind of digital mirror – one that doesn't distort, but organizes. A tool that brings structure to scattered thoughts. A partner that reminds you of your own words. And sometimes, that's all it takes: someone who listens, even when you yourself don't yet know what to say.

Those who reflect regularly with AI – through text or voice – often begin to hear their own inner voice more clearly. Not because AI replaces it, but because it creates space for it. You receive questions, impulses, sometimes even gentle confrontation – but always with the freedom to decide how deep you want to go.

If you're honest, you can rediscover yourself

What really matters is not the technology – but your willingness to be honest. AI can't force you to be truthful. But it can invite you. And if you accept that invitation, something unexpected happens: you begin to connect with yourself.

Many people stay on the surface. They function, they endure, they ignore. But when you dare to look deeper – with support, but without judgment – something can begin to shift. An inner tension, a rigid pattern, an old misunderstanding. And suddenly you realize:

I am more than my symptoms.

I am not my condition.

I am not broken.

And that's exactly what AI can offer: a space. Not an all-knowing advisor. Not a perfect therapist. But a companion tool that helps you reconnect with yourself.

Perhaps that is the most valuable contribution of this new technology: not to provide answers – but to guide you toward better questions.

Interesting Links and Resources

If you want to explore the topic of hemorrhoids, gut health, and holistic healing in more depth, you'll now find a surprisingly large range of information – both in books and online. This appendix contains a small selection of recommended resources that go beyond what has been covered in the main part of this book.

It starts with a few book recommendations that approach the topic from different angles: classical medical, holistic, personal, or naturopathic. Some of the books are written by people who have experienced these issues themselves; others are by professionals with a broader perspective on the connections between lifestyle, psyche, and body.

The second part includes links to websites and online articles focused on nutrition, pelvic floor training, alternative therapies, or psychological background. You'll also find recommendations for reliable sources of ointments, micronutrients, or medical supplies.

Thirdly, you'll find a small selection of videos and online talks, in which doctors, naturopaths, or experienced patients share their insights – whether on treatment options, surgical decisions, or what to do when nothing seems to help anymore.

The final section points to a few AI-powered tools for self-reflection: whether via text chat, voice recording, or journaling apps – modern artificial intelligence can serve as a calm, structured companion to help you better understand your symptoms, recognize patterns in your thoughts and behaviors, and develop new ways of self-observation.

Of course, no list is ever complete – and not every resource is right for every person. But maybe there's something here that inspires you, reassures you, or helps you move forward. Or simply gives you the quiet reminder that you're not alone with your questions.

Specialist Literature on Hemorrhoids (German)

"Below the Belt" by Renate Bruckmann

A holistic health guide for self-help with unexplained discomfort in the pelvic area. 50 color photos and 30 illustrations make the applications easy to follow at home.

Fk you, Hemorrhoids: Breaking Taboos with Health and Nutrition Tips**

Patient says: "Professor, I have hemorrhoids." The professor of surgery replies: "Dear patient, so do I." – What purpose do hemorrhoids actually serve, and how can the condition be easily relieved or even prevented?

After Hour – Your Proctologist Consultation: Everything You Need to Know About Constipation, Hemorrhoids, Anal Fissures, HPV, Colon Cancer, and Proper Hygiene

Open, honest, and unfiltered, Dr. Florian Frank explains abscesses, pilonidal sinus, prolapse, genital warts, colon cancer, and more — offering deep insights into the mechanisms of the rectum so your next trip to the bathroom becomes a pos-itive experience.

When Your Butt Needs Help – Expert Advice for Issues in the Taboo Zone: Treatment Options and Practical Help

Dr. Peter Ambe, a recognized expert in proctology with many years of experience, provides patients with essential knowledge in this guide – so there's no need to fear when things aren't going well back there.

Therapy to Go: 100 Psychotherapy Tools for More Ease in Everyday Life

This evidence-based psychology guide presents 100 helpful methods from psychotherapy in a clear, engaging, and entertaining way – easy to apply in your daily life.

All books are available through bookstores or online.

Interesting Links and Online Resources (German)

Hemorrhoids – Combating the Sitting Problem with Movement and Diet

Who talks openly about hemorrhoids? Although every second person over 50 in Germany struggles with their unpleasant or painful effects, they remain a taboo topic. This site offers comprehensive information on the causes and natural treatments of this vascular condition.

https://tinyurl.com/nh-haemorrhoiden

Hemorrhoids: Symptoms, Causes, and Home Remedies

Hemorrhoids affect millions of people. The most common symptoms are pain while sitting or during bowel movements, itching, and bleeding. Fortunately, home remedies are often very effective. This article from "Zentrum der Gesundheit" (Center for Health) provides a wealth of helpful information.

https://tinyurl.com/zdg-haemorrhoiden

Hemorrhoids – Osteopathy Can Help Without Surgery

For newly developed or smaller hemorrhoids, osteopathy may offer a solution without the need for surgery. The first goal is to relieve the circulatory congestion so that the blood can flow properly again and the hemorrhoids can recede.

https://tinyurl.com/ov-haemorrhoiden

Hemorrhoids – A Holistic View and Treatment Approach

Blockages in the blood vessels of the anal area can lead to blood congestion and varicose-like enlargement of the hemorrhoids, causing the well-known symptoms: burning, itching, discharge, bleeding... those affected know the struggle.

https://tinyurl.com/gh-haemorrhoiden

Interesting Online Videos

Hemorrhoids – A Few Words from a Holistic Perspective

Every second person in Germany has or has had hemorrhoids. Dr. Karl Hartner addresses such symptoms at their root and shares, in this brief video, a few interesting approaches from the perspective of complementary medicine.

https://youtu.be/Gdse4ilTWt0

Treating Hemorrhoids: Relieve Discomfort with These Tricks and Exercises (NO Tools Required)

Hemorrhoids are still often a taboo topic. In this video, Visna Stief shows several techniques and exercises that can be helpful for mild cases of hemorrhoids.

https://youtu.be/Row8nxLtGiU

Hemorrhoid Treatment | Medical Discussion Format

Prof. Dr. Detlef Meyer, Head of the Surgical Department at Leopoldina Hospital, discusses the taboo topic of "hemorrhoids" in this episode. Around 80% of people experience hemorrhoidal issues at some point in their lives.

https://youtu.be/zSxvnIL0oCk

Hemorrhoids: How to Treat Them and Recognize Symptoms | ARD

Trouble with hemorrhoids? Pain, constipation, and other bathroom struggles are more common than one might think—yet few talk about them. Dr. Katharina Abbing of WDR's "Servicezeit" brings the topic out of the taboo zone—in a setting most wouldn't expect.

https://youtu.be/9fB0fLwdfgU

Hemorrhoids: What to Do and When to Seek Medical Attention

How do I know if I have hemorrhoids? Can hemorrhoids go away on their own? Many people find the topic uncomfortable, which is why some prefer to ask the internet anonymously rather than speak with a doctor. Itching, oozing, and burning around the anus are typical symptoms of enlarged hemorrhoids. What can you do? Dr. Julia Fischer explains what helps with hemorrhoids.

https://youtu.be/-Z61xq5tp2s

AI Apps for Your Smartphone

Download on the App Store | GET IT ON Google Play

OpenAI ChatGPT - "The Original", GPT-3 is available for free. With GPT-4o and memory features, it provides excellent general knowledge and is well suited for self-reflection.

Claude.ai - Also highly suitable for self-reflection, with responses that feel almost therapeutic. Free to get started.

Google Gemini - Very good factual knowledge, but tends to use a more technical and neutral tone. Less suitable for personal reflection.

DeepSeek - Solid medical knowledge with a technical focus. Not ideal for emotional or reflective dialogue.

Final Words – You Are More Than Your Symptoms

If you've read this book all the way to the end, then you've already done something very important: you've opened yourself up to a topic that many people would rather avoid. And that alone is a brave first step. Because as simple as it may sound: healing doesn't begin with the perfect ointment or the right doctor – it begins with the decision to take yourself seriously.

Hemorrhoids are often more than just a local irritation. They are a symptom – a signal that something deeper might be out of balance. It could be your gut, your daily life, your body, or the way you relate to yourself. Those who view these signs not as a defect, but as an invitation to look more closely, are often rewarded with surprising insights.

It took me many years to understand that myself. Two surgeries, countless remedies, setbacks, frustration – and in the end, the realization: it's not about quickly "getting rid" of it. It's about understanding what's really going on inside me. And how I can shape my life in a way that makes me feel better. One step at a time.

Maybe you'll take from this book the impulse not to judge yourself too quickly, not to give up, and not to put all your hope into just one solution. Maybe you'll find your very own way – with the help of a good doctor, a helpful ointment, a new seat cushion, a walk, a conversation with yourself, or even with an artificial intelligence that helps you reflect.

What matters is this: you have influence. And you're allowed to trust yourself.

I sincerely hope that this book has not only given you new knowledge – but also new confidence, clarity, and a more compassionate view of your own body. Healing isn't always a straight path, but it is possible. And you are not alone.

Wishing you all the best on your journey,

Markus Schall

Index

A

B

C

D

E

F

G

H

I

J

L

M

N

O

P

S

Z